T0383079

Advanced Skin Cancer

Advanced Skin Cancer
A Case-Based Approach

Senior Editors
Debjani Sahni, MD
G. Robert Baler Endowed Professor of Dermatology
Director, Cutaneous Oncology Program
Department of Dermatology
Boston University School of Medicine

Adam Lerner, MD
Professor of Medicine
Section of Hematology/Oncology
Department of Medicine
Boston University School of Medicine

Junior Editor
Bilal Fawaz, MD
Assistant Professor of Dermatology
Department of Dermatology
Boston University School of Medicine

With a Foreword by
Rhoda M. Alani, MD
Herbert Mescon Endowed Professor and Chair
Department of Dermatology
Boston University School of Medicine
Dermatologist-in-Chief
Boston Medical Center

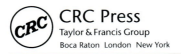

CRC Press
Taylor & Francis Group
Boca Raton London New York

CRC Press is an imprint of the
Taylor & Francis Group, an **informa** business

First edition published 2022
by CRC Press
6000 Broken Sound Parkway NW, Suite 300, Boca Raton, FL 33487-2742

and by CRC Press
4 Park Square, Milton Park, Abingdon, Oxon, OX14 4RN

ISBN: 978-0-367-13471-6 (hbk)
ISBN: 978-1-032-23024-5 (pbk)
ISBN: 978-0-429-02668-3 (ebk)

DOI: 10.1201/9780429026683

Typeset in Times
by codeMantra

Contents

Foreword

Advanced Skin Cancer: A Case-Based Approach provides case-based examples of the personalized, multidisciplinary approach to complex skin cancer management utilized at premier tertiary care cancer centers in the United States. This team-based care allows for collaborative input to inform best practices for patients with complex skin cancers. The majority of the patient cases presented in this book were seen at Boston Medical Center. As the largest safety-net hospital in New England, Boston Medical Center provides exceptional care to a diverse population of patients with unique medical needs which are often complicated by complex social determinants that greatly impact their care and outcomes. The Department of Dermatology at Boston Medical Center is the entry point for a large number of patients who present with advanced primary or metastatic skin cancers. The authors possess unique expertise in the evaluation and management of advanced cutaneous malignancies, and discuss interesting and informative cases that have presented to our dermatology care team initially, but which require a multidisciplinary approach given the complexities of cutaneous malignancy and other medical and social challenges.

The past decade has seen a tremendous expansion of personalized approaches to the treatment of cancers, with specific targeted therapies being developed for driver events in a variety of malignancies. For skin cancers, notable advances in targeted therapies for melanoma have drawn the attention of the international medical community with enthusiasm over early successes being dampened by near-universal innate or acquired resistance to such therapies. These novel therapies have been widely studied both in patients and in research laboratories, and their complex role in the management of patients with advanced melanoma continues to evolve. In addition, recent advances in the development of immunotherapies, particularly immune checkpoint inhibitors (IHIs), for a wide range of cancers have shown particular efficacy in aggressive types of cutaneous malignancies. These treatments have significantly enhanced the therapeutic armamentarium for patients with complex cutaneous malignancies and advanced disease, and are examined within the context of the cases presented here.

The unique perspectives of the editors and authors of this book have evolved from decades of clinical practice and research within complex healthcare systems which inform their decision making. This book is designed to share a pragmatic approach to complex skin cancer management that may serve as a guide for providers around the world, particularly those that care for patients with diverse social and medical needs. The text reflects state-of-the-art practices as well as team-based decision making to afford the best possible personalized care to each patient and their unique clinical and social circumstances. This book will be of particular value to any physicians caring for patients with cutaneous malignancies, either as primary care physicians or as specialty care providers. The cases presented and management through team decision making will be especially valuable to medical oncologists, surgical oncologists, dermatologists, radiation oncologists, plastic surgeons, head and neck surgeons, and nursing staff that care for patients with complex cutaneous malignancies. Case discussions will have particular relevance for physicians and advanced-practice providers who care for patients within underserved communities to demonstrate best practices when treating patients who present to healthcare providers with advanced-stage cutaneous malignancies.

Finally, the new era of personalized cancer therapeutics has also informed the critical need for a team-based approach to the treatment of patients with advanced skin cancers. Each case presented here illustrates the importance of diverse medical teams for the effective treatment of advanced skin cancers as well as the inclusion of ancillary service team members to support patients through their treatment and recovery. Such a team-based approach is particularly important in the setting of safety-net care for vulnerable populations and is critical to ensuring the best possible outcomes for these disadvantaged communities.

Rhoda M. Alani, MD
Herbert Mescon Endowed Professor and Chair
Department of Dermatology
Boston University School of Medicine
Dermatologist-in-Chief
Boston Medical Center
Boston, Massachusetts

Preface

We are fortunate to be living in a period of "oncology renaissance," an era where major advances in science and medicine have culminated in an explosion of novel therapies that are decisively making meaningful differences to the lives of cancer patients. This is certainly true for cutaneous oncology, where advanced disease states such as metastatic melanoma can finally be met with a choice of drugs that can lead to a real survival benefit in patients for whom care was previously palliative. It is becoming increasingly apparent that the most effective care of advanced cutaneous oncology patients occurs through a multidisciplinary approach utilizing evidence-based national guidelines for best practice, which considers both tumor-specific and patient-specific factors. It is discernable that there is no "one-size-fits-all" approach for the care of cutaneous oncology patients, but instead, a range of potential therapeutic options and solutions. Patient management is dictated by a combination of medical and social considerations including nuances of the cancer in question, patient co morbidities, social circumstances, access to healthcare, immediate support network, and medical healthcare coverage. Thus, the final decision in the course of management becomes personalized to each patient.

A multidisciplinary cutaneous oncology team facilitates the coordinated care between numerous specialties. This enables the appropriate expertise of each specialty to be utilized in the most effective and efficient way for the patient. A "one-stop" multidisciplinary clinic where patients can be reviewed by faculty from various specialties at the same time is more practical for the patient, while additionally allowing better communication among specialist providers, a key component of excellence in patient care. A multidisciplinary cutaneous oncology tumor board panel implements the academic review of patient- and tumor-specific factors, distinct aspects of the tumor pathology, and prevailing national guidelines to help determine the best care for patients. It also provides an important educational opportunity for trainees to observe how providers outside of their specialty arrive at decisions in patient care.

The series of cases in this book reflects the coordinated care and expertise of the multidisciplinary cutaneous oncology team at Boston Medical Center, including a chapter dedicated to patients with Merkel cell cancer managed by the cutaneous oncology team from the University of Washington Medical Center. The editors aim to illustrate the relevant contributions from each of the specialties that culminate in the final decision plan for each patient.

Debjani Sahni
Adam Lerner
Bilal Fawaz

Acknowledgments

All three editors wish to thank Rhoda Alani, MD, Chair of the Boston University School of Medicine, Department of Dermatology, for her foresight and support in the development of the Cutaneous Oncology Program in which most of the patients described in this book were seen. We are grateful to her for proposing the composition of this book and for advocating for us throughout this mammoth task.

I am fortunate to work with a highly skilled and supportive group of colleagues, the multidisciplinary cutaneous oncology team at Boston Medical Center. I would not be able to deliver excellent care to our patients without them, and they graciously contributed their talent to the book. At the start of this project, it became quickly apparent that I could not showcase the work in this book without inviting and equally involving Adam Lerner, MD, who co-manages complex patients with me. His guidance and mentorship have been invaluable. It is fortuitous that we both think alike in our patient care, but more importantly, that we listen to each other. Similarly, it would have been impossible to produce this book without the cooperation of an intelligent, organized, and patient colleague, Bilal Fawaz, MD. He was essentially my right-hand man for this task.

My final words of acknowledgment go to my family, in particular, my parents, brother, and sister who have been a part of my journey throughout. Most importantly, I am grateful to my husband Anik, and my two daughters, Sophia and Neve, who have been so patient and supportive and made everything worthwhile.

Debjani Sahni, MD

Dr. Lerner would like to acknowledge the support of his family throughout his career as an oncologist, particularly his wife, Beth Warach.

Adam Lerner, MD

I have to start by thanking my parents, Hussein and Hana, for their endless support, not only through my fellowship, but throughout my entire educational endeavor. I couldn't have done it without you.

I would also like to thank my outstanding mentors, Dr. Sahni, Dr. Lerner, and Dr. Alani, for providing me with this opportunity. This experience was invaluable in my personal and professional development.

Bilal Fawaz, MD

Editors

Debjani Sahni, MD, is the G. Robert Baler Endowed Professor and Director of the multidisciplinary Cutaneous Oncology Program at Boston University School of Medicine and Boston Medical Center, where she specializes in the medical management of advanced skin cancers. She completed her medical school training at the United Medical and Dental Schools of Guy's and St Thomas' Hospitals in London, UK. After acquiring membership of the Royal College of Physicians (MRCP), she completed her dermatology residency at the St John's Institute of Dermatology in London. She subsequently undertook a cutaneous oncology fellowship at Dana-Farber Cancer Institute and Brigham and Women's Hospital, Harvard Medical School, Boston. Dr Sahni serves as the Director of the Cutaneous Oncology Fellowship Program and the Director of the unique and highly respected International Graduate Program in Dermatology (IGPD). First established in 1988, the IGPD offers international postgraduate doctors the opportunity to train in dermatology, utilizing state-of-the-art facilities and therapies available in the United States. Her academic interests include teaching and mentoring for which she is the recipient of several teaching awards and an external examiner for postgraduate dermatology training exams internationally. Dr Sahni's clinical research interests focus on the epidemiology and treatment of skin cancers, and she is the author of multiple scientific papers, and editor and co-author for the dermatology textbook, *Melanoma in Clinical Practice*.

Adam Lerner, MD, is a Professor in the Section of Hematology/Oncology, Department of Medicine, at Boston University School of Medicine and Boston Medical Center. His clinical practice focuses on the care of patients with cutaneous and hematologic malignancies as well as sarcomas. His research focuses on cyclic nucleotide phosphodiesterase and focal adhesion complex signaling in human cancer biology.

Bilal Fawaz, MD, is an Assistant Professor in the Department of Dermatology at Boston University School of Medicine and Boston Medical Center. His notable contributions to research have been in cutaneous oncology, specifically revolving around optimizing patient outcomes and quality of life. He is the recipient of the American Society for Dermatologic Surgery's Cutting-Edge Research Grant in 2018 for his work on improving the quality of life for patients with skin cancer. He is the author of several book chapters in well-known dermatology textbooks such as *Treatment of Skin Disease* and *Melanoma in Clinical Practice*.

Contributors

Ali Al-Haseni, MD
Department of Dermatology
Boston University School of Medicine
Boston, Massachusetts

Sara Al Janahi, MD, MSc
Department of Dermatology
Boston University School of Medicine
Boston, Massachusetts

Michael R. Cassidy, MD
Department of Surgery
Division of Surgical Oncology
Boston University School of Medicine
Boston, Massachusetts

Malathi Chittireddy, MD, MSc
Department of Dermatology
Boston University School of Medicine
Boston, Massachusetts

Emily Coleman, MD
Department of Dermatology
Boston University School of Medicine
Boston, Massachusetts

Yasin Damji, MD
Department of Dermatology
Boston University School of Medicine
Boston, Massachusetts

Michael A. Dyer, MD
Department of Radiation Oncology
Boston Medical Center
Boston University School of Medicine
Boston, Massachusetts

Heather A. Edwards, MD
Department of Otolaryngology – Head and Neck
    Surgery
Boston University School of Medicine
Boston, Massachusetts

Waleed Ezzat, MD, FACS
Plastic and Reconstructive Surgery
Department of Otolaryngology – Head and Neck
    Surgery
Boston University School of Medicine
Boston, Massachusetts

Daniel L. Faden, MD, FACS
Department of Otolaryngology – Head and Neck
    Surgery
Harvard Medical School
and
Massachusetts Eye and Ear
Massachusetts General Hospital
Boston, Massachusetts

Bilal Fawaz, MD
Department of Dermatology
Boston University School of Medicine
Boston, Massachusetts

Allene Fonseca, MD
Department of Dermatology
University of Washington
Seattle, Washington

Sarah Ann Kam, MD
Department of Dermatology
Boston University School of Medicine
Boston, Massachusetts

Iman Fatima Khan, MS, MPH
Boston University School of Medicine
Boston, Massachusetts

Hannah Kopelman, DO
Department of Dermatology
Boston University School of Medicine
Boston, Massachusetts

Adam Lerner, MD
Section of Hematology/Oncology
Department of Medicine
Boston University School of Medicine
Boston, Massachusetts

Hannah E. Mumber, BS
Boston University School of Medicine
Boston, Massachusetts

Paul Nghiem, MD, PhD
Department of Dermatology
University of Washington
Fred Hutchinson Cancer Research Center
Seattle, Washington

Bichchau Michelle Nguyen, MD, MPH
Department of Dermatology
Boston University School of Medicine
Boston, Massachusetts

Connor O'Boyle, MD
Massachusetts Eye and Ear
Massachusetts General Hospital
Harvard Medical School
Boston, Massachusetts

Song Park, MD
Division of Dermatology
University of Washington
Seattle, Washington

Shreya Patel, MD
Department of Dermatology
Boston University School of Medicine
Boston, Massachusetts

Nicole Patzelt, MD
Department of Dermatology
Boston University School of Medicine
Boston, Massachusetts

Sarah Phillips, MD
Department of Dermatology
Boston University School of Medicine
Boston, Massachusetts

Elizabeth T. Rotrosen, AB
Boston University School of Medicine
Boston, Massachusetts

Tatchai Ruangrattanatavorn, MD, MSc
Department of Dermatology
Boston University School of Medicine
Boston, Massachusetts

Teviah E. Sachs, MD, MPH
Department of Surgery
Division of Surgical Oncology
Boston University School of Medicine
Boston, Massachusetts

Debjani Sahni, MD
Department of Dermatology
Boston University School of Medicine
Boston, Massachusetts

Monica Rosales Santillan, MD
Department of Dermatology
Boston University School of Medicine
Boston, Massachusetts

Shawn Shih, MD
Department of Dermatology
Boston University School of Medicine
Boston, Massachusetts

Marguerite Sullivan, MD
Department of Dermatology
Boston University School of Medicine
Boston, Massachusetts

Minh T. Truong, MD
Department of Radiation Oncology
Boston University School of Medicine
Boston, Massachusetts

1

Melanoma

Ali Al-Haseni and Debjani Sahni

CONTENTS

Introduction

Melanoma is a skin cancer originating from melanocytes that are most commonly located in the skin. Melanoma can less commonly also arise from the eye or mucosal surfaces of the head and neck, urogenital tract, and gastrointestinal surfaces.[1] Melanoma is responsible for more than 90% of deaths related to skin cancer, with incidence increasing by 270% from 1973 to 2002 in the United States.[2,3]

Epidemiology

The incidence of melanoma has been increasing steadily by 3%–4% annually.[2] The estimated current lifetime risk of melanoma in the United States is 1 in 63, with an incidence rate of 20.1 per 100,000 persons for the period between 2003 and 2007. This compares to 41.1–55.8 per 100,000 persons in Australia.[3] This increased incidence over the past five decades has been attributed to multiple factors, including increased exposure to ultraviolet (UV) radiation from sun or tanning bed use and enhanced screening leading to increased diagnosis.[2] Melanoma tends to affect middle-aged adults, with a median age of 57 years at diagnosis. In young adults (<55 years), it is more common in females, representing the sixth most common cancer in women, while for adults over the age of 55 years, it is seen more commonly in males, constituting the fifth most common cancer in men.[3,4]

DOI: 10.1201/9780429026683-1

Pathogenesis and Risk Factors

Melanoma is a multifactorial disease that results from the interaction of environmental factors in genetically predisposed individuals.[3] It is associated with a high somatic mutation burden when compared to many other human cancers. However, most of these mutations eventually lead to activation of two main pathways: The mitogen-activated protein kinase (MAPK) and the phosphoinositol-3 kinase (PI3K/AKT) pathways. MAPK is responsible for cellular proliferation, differentiation, and survival, while PI3K is responsible for cellular homeostasis. Approximately 90% of all melanomas show MAPK pathway activation. The most common mutation in the MAPK pathway is a mutation in the *BRAF* gene, with 80%–90% of the mutations being a missense mutation resulting in valine to glutamate substitution (V600E). This mutation is found in ~40%–60% of melanomas arising in intermittently sun-exposed skin. The second most common mutation in the MAPK pathway is an activating mutation in *NRAS* found in 15%–30% of melanomas, followed by *neurofibromin* 1 (NF1) tumor-suppressor gene mutation, present in 10%–15% of melanomas. However, *NF1* mutations are usually associated with chronic sun exposure.[4] The receptor tyrosine kinase *KIT* mutations are found in 2%–8% of melanomas and are usually present in acral melanomas and in melanomas arising from intermittent sun exposure. A number of other gene mutations are involved in melanoma development; some examples include *telomerase reverse transcriptase* (*TERT*) promoter mutations, *cyclin-dependent kinase inhibitor-2A* (*CDKN2A*) mutations, and *phosphatase and tensin homolog* (*PTEN*) mutations.[4]

The most important environmental risk factor for the development of melanoma is UV radiation from sun light.[3,4] Specifically, intense intermittent sun exposure (sun burns) carries a higher melanoma risk when compared with chronic continuous exposure. Other risk factors include fair skin type, red hair, blue eyes, numerous freckles, UV-A exposure (therapeutic or tanning bed use), immune suppression, multiple melanocytic nevi, and a personal or family history of melanoma.[3,4] The white population has a tenfold higher risk of developing cutaneous melanoma when compared with people of color (Black, Asian, or Hispanics). However, the rate of acral melanoma, which is not correlated with UV damage, is equal between Whites and Blacks (though it is the most common subtype of melanoma in the Black population). In the case of non-cutaneous melanomas (i.e., mucosal melanoma), although higher numbers are detected in the white population, they make up a higher proportion of melanoma subtype in patients of color compared to Whites.[5] There is a sevenfold increased risk of melanoma in patients with more than 100 melanocytic nevi, 32-fold increased risk with more than 10 atypical nevi, and 2%–5% increased risk with large congenital nevi (>20 cm in size). Despite this, only 25%–30% of melanomas arise from pre-existing nevi, with the vast majority occurring *de novo* on normal skin.[3,4,6–8] Familial cases are rare and are usually related to mutations in *CDKN2A* or *cyclin-dependent kinase-4* (*CDK4*).[3,4]

Clinical Presentation and Histological Subtypes

Melanoma presents classically as a changing brown, black, or pink pigmented skin lesion. If left untreated, it can ulcerate and/or bleed. The education campaigns targeted for early melanoma recognition by physicians and the public launched the "ABCD" criteria in 1985, with subsequent addition of the letter "E". They stand for **A**symmetry, **B**order irregularity, **C**olor variation, **D**iameter > 6 mm, and **E**volution. This can help patients considerably during regular self-skin exams, which has a sensitivity of 57%–90% for melanoma detection. Dermatoscopic findings of an atypical pigment network, irregular dots/globules/streaks, regression, or blue-white veil raise the suspicion of melanoma.[3] Melanomas are most commonly located on the back of men and the legs of women. The mortality rate of melanoma showed an initial increase of 1.4% annually between 1977 and 1990. However, a downtrend of 0.3% annually was subsequently observed for the period between 1990 and 2002.[3]

Historically, cutaneous melanomas were divided into several subtypes based on clinical factors or histopathological growth patterns. *Superficial spreading melanoma* accounts for 70% of cases with an early radial growth phase in the epidermis followed by a vertical growth phase in the dermis. *Nodular melanoma*, which accounts for 5% of cases, presents as a rapidly growing, often ulcerating, brown-black nodule which has a vertical growth pattern from the outset with no radial growth pattern. Nodular melanoma is associated with an aggressive biological behavior. *Lentigo maligna melanoma* accounts for 4%–15% of melanomas arising in chronically sun-exposed areas (head and neck). This subtype has a very prolonged radial growth phase with slow growth over years before invading the papillary dermis. *Acral lentiginous melanoma* accounts for 5% of cases in Whites but represents the most common subtype of melanoma in people of color. This subtype arises on the palms, soles, digits, and nails. *Desmoplastic melanoma* typically appears as a pink or pale scar-like papule that is characterized histologically by an infiltrative growth pattern and frequent perineural invasion. The term *amelanotic melanoma* is often used to describe melanomas lacking dark brown-black pigmentation on clinical exam, but does not specify any histological or clinical subtype.[3,9] These clinicopathological descriptive subtypes of melanoma are slowly being phased out in favor of a molecular description for melanoma, for example, *BRAF*-positive melanoma and c-KIT-positive melanoma. The latter subclassification provides more valuable information regarding the origin of the cancer and the possible therapeutic options, which is more meaningful in clinical practice.[10]

Treatment and Prognosis

Most cases of melanoma are diagnosed early, and therefore, surgical excision is usually the first-line treatment for achieving cure in the majority of cases. Some cases, however, subsequently relapse with local recurrence or regional/distant metastasis. Approximately 10% of melanoma cases present with unresectable disease due to regional or metastatic disease at the time of diagnosis.[4] The National Comprehensive Cancer Network (NCCN) recommends wide local excision of melanomas with 1 cm margins if the primary tumor is equal to or less than 1 mm in thickness, 1–2 cm margins if the primary tumor is >1–2 mm in thickness, and 2 cm margins for all melanomas thicker than 2 mm. The addition of sentinel lymph node biopsy (SLNB) is recommended for tumors equal to or more than 0.8 mm in thickness or for tumors less than 0.8 mm in thickness if ulceration is noticed on histopathology.[11,12]

Until recently, treatment of metastatic melanoma was mostly palliative with chemotherapy and/or radiation. Since 2011, the approval of several targeted therapies and immune checkpoint inhibitors has revolutionized the field of melanoma therapeutics and significantly improved the survival of metastatic melanoma patients.[13] Agents used for targeted therapy include BRAF inhibitors (e.g., dabrafenib) and MEK inhibitors (e.g., trametinib). Immune checkpoint inhibitor therapeutic agents include cytotoxic T-lymphocyte-associated antigen-4 (CTLA-4) inhibitors (e.g., ipilimumab) and programmed cell death 1 (PD-1) inhibitors (e.g., pembrolizumab).[4] Other recently approved modalities include Talimogene Laherparepvec (T-VEC), which is a modified oncolytic herpes simplex virus type 1 (HSV-1) having the capacity to express granulocyte macrophage colony-stimulating factor (GM-CSF). T-VEC is approved as intralesional therapy for use in inoperable metastases that are accessible to injection.[13,14]

References

1. Al-Haseni A, Vrable A, Mathews S, et al. Survival outcomes of mucosal melanoma in the USA. *Futur Oncol.* 2019; 15(34): 3977–3986. doi:10.2217/fon-2019-0465.
2. Gardner LJ, Strunck JL, Wu YP, et al. Current controversies in early-stage melanoma: questions on incidence, screening, and histologic regression. *J Am Acad Dermatol.* 2019; 80(1): 1–12. doi:10.1016/j.jaad.2018.03.053.
3. Rastrelli M, Tropea S, Rossi CR, et al. Melanoma: epidemiology, risk factors, pathogenesis, diagnosis and classification. *In Vivo.* 2014; 28(6): 1005–1012. https://pubmed-ncbi-nlm-nih-gov.ezproxy.bu.edu/25398793/. Accessed September 7, 2020.
4. Leonardi GC, Falzone L, Salemi R, et al. Cutaneous melanoma: from pathogenesis to therapy (review). *Int J Oncol.* 2018; 52(4): 1071–1080. doi:10.3892/ijo.2018.4287.
5. Rigel DS. Epidemiology of melanoma. *Semin Cutan Med Surg.* 2010; 29(4): 204–209. doi:10.1016/j.sder.2010.10.005.

6. Gandini S, Sera F, Cattaruzza MS, et al. Meta-analysis of risk factors for cutaneous melanoma: I. Common and atypical naevi. *Eur J Cancer*. 2005; 41(1): 28–44. doi:10.1016/j.ejca.2004.10.015.

7. Watt AJ, Kotsis SV, Chung KC. Risk of melanoma arising in large congenital melanocytic nevi: a systematic review. *Plast Reconstr Surg*. 2004; 113(7): 1968–1974. doi:10.1097/01.PRS.0000122209.10277.2A.

8. Tucker M, Halpern A, Holly E, et al. Clinically recognized dysplastic nevi. A central risk factor for cutaneous melanoma, *JAMA*. 1997; 277(18): 1439–1444. PubMed: https://pubmed.ncbi.nlm.nih.gov/9145715/. Accessed September 7, 2020.

9. Wee E, Wolfe R, Mclean C, et al. Clinically amelanotic or hypomelanotic melanoma: anatomic distribution, risk factors, and survival. *J Am Acad Dermatol*. 2018; 79(4): 645.e4–651.e4. doi:10.1016/j.jaad.2018.04.045.

10. Rabbie R, Ferguson P, Molina-Aguilar C, et al. Melanoma subtypes: genomic profiles, prognostic molecular markers and therapeutic possibilities. *J Pathol*. 2019; 247(5): 539–551. doi:10.1002/path.5213.

11. NCCN. National Comprehensive Cancer Network (NCCN). https://www.nccn.org/professionals/physician_gls/pdf/nmsc.pdf. Accessed August 15, 2020.

12. Faries MB, Thompson JF, Cochran AJ, et al. Completion dissection or observation for sentinel-node metastasis in melanoma. *N Engl J Med*. 2017; 376(23): 2211–2222. doi:10.1056/NEJMoa1613210.

13. Terheyden P, Krackhardt A, Eigentler T. The systemic treatment of melanoma. The place of immune checkpoint inhibitors and the suppression of intracellular signal transduction. *Dtsch Arztebl Int*. 2019; 116(29–30): 497–504. doi:10.3238/arztebl.2019.0497.

14. Perez MC, Miura JT, Naqvi SMH, et al. Talimogene Laherparepvec (TVEC) for the treatment of advanced melanoma: a single-institution experience. *Ann Surg Oncol*. 2018; 25(13): 3960–3965. doi:10.1245/s10434-018-6803-0.

Case 1.1

Authors: Nicole Patzelt, MD, Malathi Chittireddy, MD, MSc, Hannah E. Mumber, BS, and Adam Lerner, MD.

Reason for Presentation: Management of a melanoma patient with regional lymph node metastases.

Chief Complaint: Growth on the left arm.

History of Present Illness: A middle-aged woman presented to the dermatology clinic for evaluation of a growth on the left upper extremity. The patient first noted the lesion shortly after the primary care provider removed another lesion in the same area 1 year prior to this presentation. The lesion began as a small asymptomatic "spot" that enlarged gradually over the year. More recently, it started to drain yellow fluid. The patient grew up with a "beach lifestyle" and reported several blistering sunburns during childhood as well as the frequent use of tanning beds.

Review of Systems: Denied weight loss, enlarged lumps in the neck, axillae, and groin areas. Denied headaches or dizziness.

Medical/Surgical History: Nil relevant.

Medications: Nil relevant.

Family History: Sister had several basal cell carcinomas.

Physical Examination: Fitzpatrick skin type II; Left upper arm: A 2 cm ulcerated, pink nodule, draining yellow discharge; the borders were raised (see Figure 1.1.1), and it was tender on palpation; no palpable lymphadenopathy in the cervical, axillary, or inguinal areas.

Pathology: Left upper arm, punch biopsy (see Figure 1.1.2): (A) Irregular aggregates of atypical squamous epithelium. The melanocytic proliferation is difficult to appreciate at low power (H&E, 40×). (B) Higher power reveals atypical melanocytes arranged in nests (H&E, 400×). (C) The melanocytes are positive with immunoperoxidase staining for SOX-10 (400×). Consistent with malignant melanoma arising in association with squamous cell carcinoma (SCC).

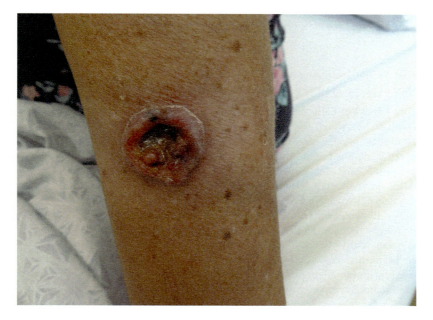

FIGURE 1.1.1 Ulcerated nodule on the left upper arm.

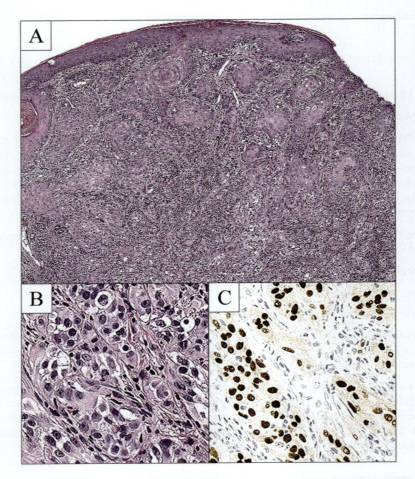

FIGURE 1.1.2 Punch biopsy from the left upper arm nodule: (A) H&E, low power; (B) H&E, high power; and (C) SOX-10 immunostain.

Final Diagnosis: Melanoma arising in association with SCC; Breslow thickness of 2.2 mm, Clark Level IV, with presence of ulceration and 8 mitoses/mm^2; Stage II (T3b, NxMx); *BRAF* mutation negative.

Management and Disease Course: Based on NCCN guidelines, the patient underwent a 2 cm wide local excision with SLNB, which revealed 4/9 positive lymph nodes. This upstaged her to stage III (T3b, N3, M0). The multidisciplinary tumor board panel advised active nodal basin surveillance with regular US imaging every 3 months based on data from the Multicenter Selective Lymphadenectomy Trial II (MSLT-II). In addition, adjuvant immunotherapy was recommended as per the NCCN guidelines. The patient was started on nivolumab 480 mg IV every 28 days.

After eight cycles of nivolumab, a repeat PET/CT CAP and brain MRI showed multiple new metastases in the subcutaneous tissues of the trunk, supraclavicular, submandibular, parotid, and inguinal regions, as well as several brain metastases. This new data upstaged the patient to stage IV (T3b, N3, M1).

The patient underwent Cyberknife treatment for the largest brain metastasis, which was well tolerated. Given the brain metastases and overall progressive disease, the patient was commenced on dual checkpoint inhibitor immunotherapy by adding ipilimumab to nivolumab. This subsequently led to a rapid and durable complete response to the combined therapy, with resolution of both the central nervous system (CNS) and subcutaneous metastases.

Discussion

- The Multicenter Selective Lymphadenectomy Trials (MSLT-I and MSLT-II) are two well-known pivotal studies that helped elucidate which patients with melanoma would benefit clinically from a SLNB, and whether there is a survival benefit of pursuing completion lymph node dissection (CLND) in patients who are sentinel node positive. Based on the results of these studies, guidelines have been developed to avoid patients getting unnecessary and potentially morbid surgical procedures that have no proven survival benefit.

- MSLT-I was a phase III trial published in 2014 by Morton et al. The authors evaluated 2001 patients with primary cutaneous melanoma. They were randomly assigned to undergo wide local excision of the primary melanoma with subsequent nodal observation and complete lymphadenectomy for any nodal relapse versus wide local excision with SLNB and immediate complete lymphadenectomy if nodal metastases were detected on biopsy.[1,2]

- Overall survival (OS) was not affected significantly by the treatment itself, with 81.4% survival in the biopsy group and 78.3% survival in the observation group. The mean 10-year disease-free survival rates, however, were significantly improved in the biopsy group compared to the observation group for patients with intermediate-thickness (1.2–3.5 mm) or thick (>3.5 mm) melanoma. Specifically, rates were 71.3%±1.8% compared to 64.7%±2.3% for intermediate-thickness melanoma and 50.7%±4.0% versus 40.5%±4.7% for thick melanoma.[2]

- In patients with intermediate-thickness melanoma undergoing SLNB, the 10-year distant disease-free survival rate, as well as the 10-year melanoma-specific survival rate, was improved. The hazard ratio for distant metastasis was 0.62 and for death from melanoma was 0.56.[2]

- Based on this study, SLNB was recommended for staging of all intermediate and thick primary cutaneous melanomas. This would help identify patients at greater risk of disease recurrence and enable appropriate selection for trials in advanced melanoma. Based on the standard of care at the time of the trial, all patients with nodal metastases noted on SLNB were considered for CLND.[2]

- MSLT-II was a phase III trial published in 2017 by Faries et al. They evaluated 1934 patients with melanoma who had biopsy-proven sentinel-node metastasis. They were randomly assigned to undergo CLND versus nodal observation with ultrasonography. The objective was to evaluate the usefulness of CLND for these patients as it had been noted in MSLT-I that 88% of patients with a single sentinel-node metastasis have no additional nodal metastases after the CLND specimen is fully examined.[1,3]

- The results showed that mean 3-year melanoma-specific survival rates were not significantly different in the CLND group as compared to the observation group. Rates were 86%±1.3% and 86%±1.2%, respectively. Although non-sentinel-node metastases were only found in 11.5% of patients in the CLND group, this was noted to be a strong, independent prognostic factor for melanoma recurrence.[3]

- In the CLND group, the disease-free survival rate was slightly higher at 3 years with an increased rate of disease control in the regional nodes at 3 years. This higher rate of regional disease control was also associated with greater complications; 24.1% of patients in the CLND group developed lymphedema compared to 6.3% of patients in the observation group.[3]

- Based on this study, the value of CLND was deemed controversial. It was shown to improve regional disease control and provide prognostic information for the likelihood of melanoma recurrence. However, it did not increase melanoma-specific survival in patients with melanoma and sentinel-node metastases, and it was associated with a greater rate of complications.[3]

Teaching Pearls

- SLNB is recommended as a staging procedure for all patients with intermediate-thickness and thick primary cutaneous melanomas based on the findings of the MSLT-I.
- The value of CLND is more controversial. CLND provides no survival benefit but improves regional disease control. However, this is at the expense of a higher complication risk, including lymphedema.
- The decision of whether to pursue CLND requires a case-by-case evaluation, taking into account patient-specific factors and logistics.

References

1. Morton, DL. Overview and update of the phase III multicenter selective lymphadenectomy trials (MSLT-I and MSLT-II) in melanoma. *Clin Exp Metastasis*. 2012; 29(7): 699–706.
2. Morton D, Thompson J, Cochran A, et al. Final trial report of sentinel-node biopsy versus nodal observation in melanoma. *N Engl J Med*. 2014; 370(7): 599–609.
3. Faries M, Thompson J, Cochran A, et al. Complete dissection or observation for sentinel-node metastasis in melanoma. *N Engl J Med*. 2017; 376: 2211–2222.

Case 1.2

Authors: Marguerite Sullivan, MD, Tatchai Ruangrattanatavorn, MD, MSc, Elizabeth T. Rotrosen, AB, and Teviah E. Sachs, MD, MPH.

Reason for Presentation: Approach to an SLNB-positive patient.

Chief Complaint: Changing mole of the left upper thigh.

History of Present Illness: A young patient presented to an outside dermatologist for evaluation of an enlarging, changing mole on the left upper thigh of over 1-year duration. More recently, it had started to itch and bleed. There was a history of severe, blistering childhood sunburns.

Review of Systems: No pertinent positives.

Medical/Surgical History: None.

Medications: None.

Family History: No family history of skin cancer.

Social History: 30+ pack-year history of tobacco use; denied alcohol or illicit drug use.

Physical Exam: Fitzpatrick skin type I; left upper anterior thigh: 1.5 cm exophytic brown verrucous nodule with central hemorrhagic crust and a wide pigmented plaque at the base (see Figure 1.2.1).

Pathology: Left upper anterior thigh, shave biopsy (see Figure 1.2.2): (A) Verrucous tumor with epidermal and dermal components (H&E, 10×). (B) Higher power demonstrating nested and single hyperchromatic melanocytes in the epidermis and filling the papillary dermis (H&E, 200×). (C) Tumor cells are positive with immunoperoxidase staining for Mart-1 (200×). Consistent with malignant melanoma.

Melanoma pathologic stage T4bNxMx (at least 5.1 mm thickness, lesion extends to deep margins, ulceration present, 6/mm^2 mitoses, tumor infiltrating lymphocytes present, vascular invasion suspected, no regression).

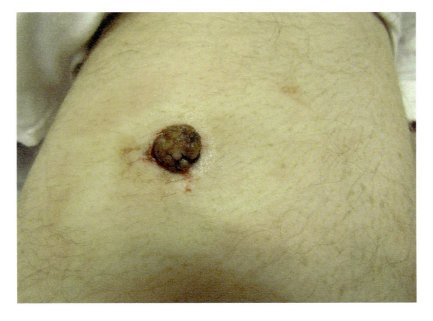

FIGURE 1.2.1 Pigmented ulcerated nodule on the left upper anterior thigh.

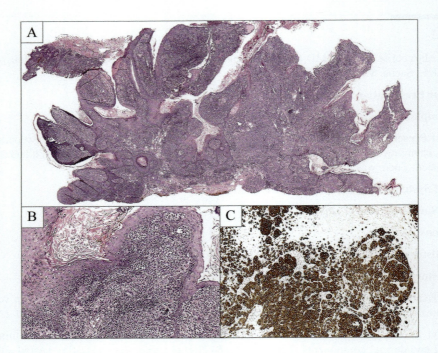

FIGURE 1.2.2   Shave biopsy of the left upper anterior thigh nodule: (A) H&E, low power; (B) H&E, high power; and (C) MART-1 immunostain.

Final Diagnosis: Melanoma at least stage IIb, AJCC (Eighth Edition) pathologic stage: T4bNxMx.

Management and Disease Course: According to the NCCN guidelines, the patient underwent wide local excision (WLE) and SLNB. Two sentinel lymph nodes were identified, both of which returned positive for a melanoma yielding a final pathologic stage IIIc (pT4bpN2aMX). Subsequent staging whole-body FDG PET-CT and brain MRI did not show any evidence of distant metastases.

For stage III patients, the NCCN guidelines recommend either nodal observation or CLND in addition to adjuvant therapy. Multidisciplinary tumor board discussion yielded a consensus that the patient should not undergo CLND but have short-interval follow-up and serial monitoring with regular clinical examination and regional ultrasound every 4 months for the first 2 years and every 6 months for the subsequent 3 years. Further testing confirmed his tumor to be PD-L1 negative and *BRAF V600E* mutation positive. The patient was given adjuvant nivolumab monotherapy for 1 year with no evidence of disease recurrence to date.

Discussion

- The MSLT-I and MSLT-II are two pivotal trials that have helped clinicians determine the best approach in managing regional lymph nodes in melanoma patients. Based on the MSLT-II trial, the value of performing a CLND for all patients with nodal metastases found on SLNB was questioned. It was shown to increase the rate of regional disease control and provide prognostic information for recurrence of melanoma but did not increase melanoma-specific survival in these patients. The likely reason for this is that most patients with nodal metastases had all their nodal metastases removed during the SLNB, and therefore, no additional therapeutic value could be derived from a CLND. Based on these findings, the NCCN guidelines recommend adjuvant systemic therapy with active nodal basin surveillance with ultrasound rather than CLND for patients with nodal metastases noted on SLNB.[1]

- Adjuvant therapy is generally recommended for AJCC stage III which entails regional spread of melanoma without distant metastases. The decision to recommend adjuvant therapy after surgery for melanoma is based on the risk of systemic relapse of the melanoma. It is worth noting that the prognosis for stage III disease is heterogeneous. The 5-year melanoma-specific survival ranges from 78% in stage IIIa disease to 40% in stage IIIc disease (AJCC Seventh Edition). Even at the microscopic level, patients who are stage IIIA with <1 mm tumor burden in the sentinel node have a 10-year melanoma-specific mortality of less than 10%. The decision of adjuvant therapy versus observation, therefore, needs to consider the risk-benefit ratio of the drug in question with the prognosis of the disease stage itself.[2]

- The first drug to receive Food and Drug Administration (FDA) approval in the adjuvant setting of melanoma was high-dose ipilimumab 10 mg/kg following a randomized control trial where the alternate arm was placebo. The drug approval came after demonstration of an improved 3-year recurrence-free survival (RFS), distant metastasis-free survival, and OS in the ipilimumab arm versus the placebo arm [65.4% versus 54.4%; hazard ratio (HR) for death 0.72; 95.1% confidence interval (CI) 0.58–0.88; $P = 0.001$]. However, this drug is no longer recommended in the adjuvant setting for melanoma in the current NCCN guidelines due to its association with severe toxicities that led to discontinuation of the drug in >80% of patients, as well as treatment-related death in five of the trial patients.[3]

- Ipilimumab in the adjuvant setting has been replaced by PD-1 inhibitors nivolumab and pembrolizumab, both of which have shown greater efficacy and tolerability. In the CheckMate-238 trial, patients with stage IIIB-C and stage IV resected melanoma treated with nivolumab demonstrated greater RFS than those in the ipilimumab arm (HR 0.71; 95% CI 0.60–0.86, $P = 0.0003$). The benefit was seen in all stage subtypes and was independent of *BRAF* mutation status.[4] In the KEYNOTE-054 trial, adjuvant pembrolizumab significantly improved RFS compared with placebo (HR 0.59; 95% CI 0.49–0.70). This was in addition to improved distant metastasis-free survival, especially in patients who were *BRAF* positive (HR 0.51) and PDL-1 negative (HR 0.45). The KEYNOTE-054 trial excluded stage IV patients and those with in-transit metastasis, but unlike the prior trial, it included patients who were stage IIIA (with SLN disease > 1 mm).[5]

- In patients with *BRAF*-mutant melanoma, the option of using combination targeted therapy is available in addition to immune checkpoint therapy. The COMBI-AD trial compared the effects of combination dabrafenib and trametinib with placebo in patients who had *BRAF* mutation-positive melanoma inclusive of stage IIIA (SLN disease > 1 mm) and stage IIIB-C. The combination therapy arm did better than the placebo arm with regard to 3-year RFS (58% versus 39%) and OS (86% and 77%). In the 5-year updated study, the RFS was confirmed across all subtypes of stage III disease [HR (95% CI): IIIA, 0.61 (0.35–1.07); IIIB, 0.50 (0.37–0.67); IIIC, 0.48 (0.36–0.64)].[6]

- Although the efficacy of the above-mentioned adjuvant therapies has been demonstrated in clinical trials, a few points are worth noting. None of the above trials included patients with stage IIIA (SLN disease < 1 mm) melanoma, and the CheckMate-238 did not include patients with stage IIIA at all, so we do not really know the value of adjuvant systemic therapy in this subgroup. The AJCC (Seventh Edition) was used to stage patients in the above-mentioned trials. Thus, stage IIIA melanoma patients had a worse prognosis in the trials than what is considered stage IIIA in the current clinical practice with more recent AJCC editions. Additionally, the trial patients underwent CLND, but this is no longer the standard of practice. Our patients in clinic are, therefore, not exactly comparable to the trial patients.[7]

- Although three options exist at present for adjuvant systemic therapy in melanoma, there are no predictive biomarkers to help guide clinicians on the choice of therapy for each patient. Clinicians need to decide based on patient-specific factors such as comorbidities, age, and performance status. Though there have been no head-to-head comparisons, single-agent immunotherapy is generally associated with fewer grade 3–4 adverse events (~15%) in comparison to combination targeted therapy (~40%), and this may be used as an argument for using PD-1 inhibitor monotherapy as first-line adjuvant therapy in melanoma.[8]

Teaching Pearls

- Melanoma patients with thicker lesions and regional disease have a greater chance of disease relapse despite the initial surgical resection.
- LND is no longer the standard of care for stage III disease as it shows no improvement in OS compared to observation.
- Both immunotherapy and combination targeted therapy have demonstrated clinical benefit in the adjuvant setting with improved RFS.

References

1. Faries M, Thompson J, Cochran A, et al. Complete dissection or observation for sentinel-node metastasis in melanoma. *N Engl J Med.* 2017; 376: 2211–2222.
2. Balch C, Gershenwald J, Soong S-J, et al. Final version of 2009 AJCC melanoma staging and classification. *J Clin Oncol.* 2009; 27: 6199.
3. Eggermont AMM, Chiarion-Sileni V, Grob JJ, et al. Adjuvant ipilimumab versus placebo after complete resection of high-risk stage III melanoma (EORTC 18071): a randomised, double-blind, phase 3 trial. *Lancet Oncol.* 2015; 16: 522–530.
4. Weber J, Vecchio MD, Mandala M, et al. 1076O Adjuvant nivolumab (NIVO) vs ipilimumab (IPI) in resected stage III/IV melanoma: 4-y recurrence-free and overall survival (OS) results from CheckMate 238. *Ann Oncol.* 2020; 31: S731–S732.
5. Eggermont AMM, Blank CU, Mandala' M, et al. LBA46 Pembrolizumab versus placebo after complete resection of high-risk stage III melanoma: final results regarding distant metastasis-free survival from the EORTC 1325-MG/keynote 054 double-blinded phase III trial. *Ann Oncol.* 2020; 31: S1175.
6. Hauschild A, Dummer R, Santinami M, et al. Long-term benefit of adjuvant dabrafenib þ trametinib (DþT) in patients (pts) with resected stage III BRAF V600emutant melanoma: five-year analysis of COMBIAD. *J Clin Oncol.* 2020; 38: 10001.
7. Troiani T, De Falco V, Napolitano S, et al. How we treat locoregional melanoma. *ESMO Open.* 2021; 6(3): 100136.
8. Napolitano S, Brancaccio G, Argenziano G, et al. It is finally time for adjuvant therapy in melanoma. *Cancer Treat Rev.* 2018; 69: 101–111.

Case 1.3

Authors: Nicole Patzelt, MD, Malathi Chittireddy, MD, MSc, Hannah E. Mumber, BS, and Adam Lerner, MD.

Reason for Presentation: A case where nodal metastases of melanoma may be best approached with CLND and systemic therapy.

Chief Complaint: Changing lesion on the right leg.

History of Present Illness: An older patient presented to the cutaneous oncology clinic for evaluation of a changing pigmented mole on the right lateral shin. Although the mole had been present for over 20 years, 3 months prior to presentation, an enlarging bump developed within the mole and started to bleed. There was a history of multiple blistering childhood sunburns and frequent use of tanning beds when the patient was younger.

Review of Systems: Denied weight loss, enlarged lymph nodes, or shortness of breath.

Medical/Surgical History: Nil relevant.

Medications: None.

Family History: First-degree relatives with history of non-melanoma skin cancer.

Physical Exam: Skin type II; right shin: 2.5 × 2.0 cm dome-shaped gray exophytic nodule covered by black crust, with a thin line of brown pigment network (see Figure 1.3.1); no inguinal, axillary, or cervical lymphadenopathy.

Pathology: Incisional biopsy of the right shin nodule (see Figure 1.3.2): (A) Deeply infiltrative dermal-based tumor (H&E, 10×). (B) Higher power revealing nested atypical melanocytes (H&E, 200×). (C) Tumor cells are positive with immunoperoxidase staining for SOX-10 (400×).

Final Diagnosis: Malignant melanoma of the right shin.

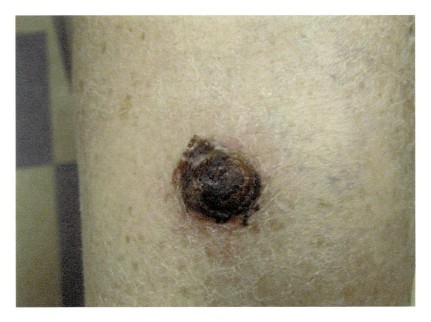

FIGURE 1.3.1   Pigmented ulcerated nodule on the right shin.

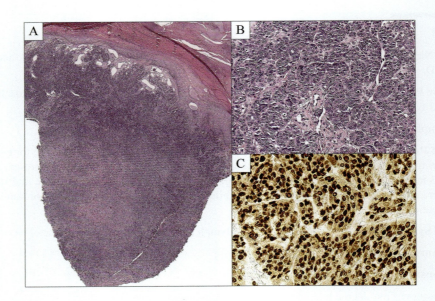

FIGURE 1.3.2   Incisional biopsy of the right shin nodule: (A) H&E, low power; (B) H&E, high power; and (C) SOX-10 immunostain.

Management and Course of Disease: One week after the skin biopsy confirmed the diagnosis of melanoma, the patient presented with a rapidly enlarging mass in the right groin suspicious for progressive inguinal adenopathy. A staging whole-body PET-CT confirmed FDG-avid right inguinal and external iliac lymphadenopathy consistent with metastatic disease. Metastatic melanoma was confirmed with ultrasound-guided biopsy, and the patient was upstaged to stage III melanoma. The multidisciplinary tumor board team recommended WLE of the primary with CLND to achieve regional disease control in this rapidly progressing melanoma, followed by adjuvant systemic therapy.

Surgery revealed metastatic melanoma in 7 out of the 18 resected lymph nodes with evidence of extranodal extension. A pelvic lymph node dissection had to be carried out at the time of CLND as the disease had further progressed here at the time of the surgery. The patient was then initiated on nivolumab monotherapy. Unfortunately, a restaging whole-body PET-CT after 3 months of nivolumab showed further disease progression to stage IV with new lesions detected in the left lung as well as the right popliteal fossa. Analysis of the resected nodal melanoma showed PDL-1 level < 1% and a *BRAF V600E* mutation.

Nivolumab was discontinued and the patient was initiated on combination targeted therapy with dabrafenib 150 mg BID and trametinib 2 mg daily. She tolerated the treatment well without any major side effects other than mild nausea. Restaging whole-body PET-CT 3 months after initiation of targeted therapy showed resolution of disease at all metastatic sites. Six months later, there was no evidence of active metastatic disease on imaging and medication was continued. The patient was then unexpectedly hospitalized with jaundice, hyperbilirubinemia, and transaminitis, thought to be related to her targeted therapy. After discontinuing those medications and resolution of her hepatitis, she was switched to vemurafenib and cobimetinib, an alternate BRAF/MEK inhibitor combination. The patient tolerated this treatment well with normal subsequent liver function tests and continued to be free of disease 14 months after initiation of BRAF/MEK inhibitor combination therapy. During the treatment course, the patient developed uveitis, a known complication of targeted therapy, which was managed with glucocorticoid eye drops by an ophthalmologist without the need to discontinue targeted therapy.

Stable disease was maintained for the next 18 months of BRAF/MEK inhibitor therapy, but eventually, the melanoma progressed with symptomatic brain metastases. Treatment was switched to combination ipilimumab/nivolumab therapy, complicated by immune checkpoint-associated colitis, and the patient ultimately succumbed to progressive CNS disease.

Discussion

- The MSLT-I and MSLT-II are two well-known studies that have helped clinicians decide which patients with melanoma are likely to benefit clinically from an SLNB or a CLND. In comparison to case 1.2 who was SLNB positive but managed with adjuvant therapy and active nodal basin surveillance with ultrasound, the current case demonstrates a situation when CLND may be indicated for select patients with nodal metastases. In a study by Reintgen et al., it was noted that disease-free survival and OS decrease if the non-sentinel lymph nodes are involved compared to only the sentinel lymph nodes.[1]

- CLND can improve local disease control, particularly in cases of bulky, clinically enlarged metastases, as in this case, where the patient developed a rapidly growing, aggressively behaving melanoma. Although lymph nodes were not palpable at the time of initial presentation, they became palpable within a week of presentation to the clinic. The rapid growth posed a risk for local deleterious effects, including pressure, necrosis, ulceration, and bleeding, which could negatively impact the patient's quality of life. Given the *BRAF* mutation and progression on monotherapy with PD-1 inhibitor, the patient was switched to targeted therapy with combination BRAF/MEK inhibitor and remained controlled for some time. However, with progression to brain metastases, therapy had to be changed again to combined immune checkpoint therapy, which is typically used as first-line therapy in this situation due to its efficacy and potential for durable response.[2] This is discussed in more detail in Case 1.4.

- Recent long-term follow-up studies have examined which subsets of patients with metastatic melanoma might benefit from combined checkpoint inhibitor therapy with both anti-CTLA-4 and anti-PD-1 therapeutics rather than monotherapy with an anti-PD-1 agent. This patient's tumor exhibited two characteristics suggestive of improved outcome with combined checkpoint inhibitor blockade. In a follow-up of the CheckMate 067 trial, addition of ipilimumab to nivolumab improved 5-year OS in *BRAF*-mutant patients from 46% to 60% (RR 0.7, 95% CI 0.46–1.05) relative to patients treated with nivolumab alone. Similarly, combined therapy also improved survival relative to anti-PD-1 monotherapy in patients whose tumor expressed a PD-L1 level less than 1% (61.4 vs. 23.5 months median OS; RR 0.69; 95% CI 0.50–0.97). In the current treatment era, serious consideration would be given to combined checkpoint inhibitor therapy in a patient with a *BRAF*-mutant and/or PD-L1-negative melanoma.[3]

Teaching Pearls

- There are instances where CLND may be indicated to achieve regional control for select patients with nodal metastases. This may include patients with clinically apparent metastatic involvement of non-sentinel lymph nodes, bulky metastases, and rapidly progressing, aggressive melanoma such as the case described.

- Although at present there are no biomarkers to predict the response of combined immune checkpoint therapy, data suggest that advanced melanoma patients with either the *BRAF* mutation or PD-L1-negative status may benefit from combined therapy with CTLA-4 and PD-1 inhibitors versus monotherapy with PD-1 inhibitor.

References

1. Reintgen M, Murray L, Akman K, et al. Evidence for a better nodal staging system for melanoma: the clinical relevance of metastatic disease confined to the sentinel lymph nodes. *Ann Surg Oncol.* 2013; 20(2): 668–674.
2. Larkin J, Chiarion-Sileni V, Gonzalez R, et al. Combined nivolumab and ipilimumab or monotherapy in untreated melanoma. *N Engl J Med.* 2015; 373(1): 23–34.
3. Larkin J, Chiarion-Sileni V, Gonzalez R, et al. Five-year survival with combined nivolumab and ipilimumab in advanced melanoma. *N Engl J Med.* 2019; 381(16): 1535–1546.

Case 1.4

Authors: Marguerite Sullivan, MD, Tatchai Ruangrattanatavorn, MD, MSc, Elizabeth T. Rotrosen, AB, and Adam Lerner, MD.

Reason for Presentation: Metastatic melanoma treated successfully with immunotherapy.

Chief Complaint: Lump on the back.

History of Present Illness: A middle-aged patient presented with a growth on his back for which he had not previously sought treatment. The lump had enlarged over 3 years. Four months prior to presentation, it had become painful and started to bleed. Around the same time, a new asymptomatic lump was noted in the right armpit.

Review of Systems: Positive for right shoulder pain and stiffness and low back pain. Negative for weight loss or other systemic symptoms.

Medical/Surgical History: Nil relevant.

Medications: Nil relevant.

Family History: No pertinent positives.

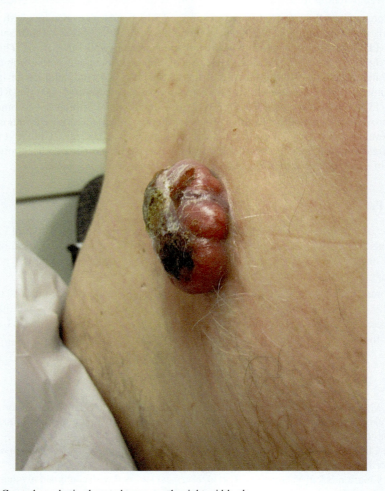

FIGURE 1.4.1   Crusted exophytic ulcerated tumor on the right mid-back.

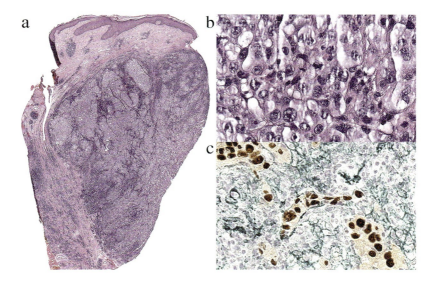

FIGURE 14.2 Incisional wedge biopsy of the right mid-back tumor: (a) H&E, low power; (b) H&E, high power; and (c) SOX-10 immunostain.

Social History: Twenty-year history of tobacco use, up to one pack per day.

Physical Examination: Fitzpatrick skin type II; Right mid-back (see Figure 1.4.1): 4.5 × 4.0 cm pink exophytic tumor with overlying hemorrhagic crust, with a background of blanching erythema surrounding the tumor; Lymph node: Three enlarged, firm, matted lymph nodes (with the largest being approximately 5 cm in diameter) were palpable in his right axilla.

Pathology: Incisional biopsy of the right mid-back (see Figure 1.4.2): (a) A deeply invasive tumor filling the dermis (H&E, 10×). (b) Higher power revealing sheet-like growth of atypical epithelioid melanocytes with occasional mitotic figures (H&E, 400×). (c) Combined immunoperoxidase staining for SOX10 and CD31 demonstrating lymphovascular invasion by melanoma cells (400×). Consistent with malignant melanoma, nodular type.

Investigations

- **Ultrasound-guided fine needle aspiration (FNA):** Of the right axillary lymph nodes confirmed malignant melanoma.
- **PET/CT:** Abnormal uptake associated with multiple enlarged right axillary lymph nodes; intense focal uptake also localized to the exophytic superficial lesion of the posterior body wall to the right of the midline below the level of the diaphragm, at about T12-L1, consistent with the patient's known primary melanoma.
- **Brain MRI:** Evidence of small multifocal-enhancing lesions throughout the bilateral cerebral hemispheres.

Diagnosis: Malignant melanoma with metastasis to the right axillary lymph nodes and multiple metastases to the brain; stage IV disease.

Management: According to the NCCN guidelines, the patient underwent WLE and CLND. Regarding the brain metastases, the cutaneous oncology tumor board panel opted to avoid whole brain radiation due to the morbidity associated with this, in particular, the risk of memory loss and poor brain function in an otherwise, young and healthy individual. Instead, the panel opted to start combined immunotherapy with anti-PD-1 and anti-CTLA-4 immune checkpoint inhibitors.

After two cycles of combined nivolumab and ipilimumab therapy, the patient developed grade 1 transaminitis and grade 3 colitis, which warranted withholding treatment and starting a prednisone taper. Three weeks later, the colitis and transaminitis resolved and nivolumab as monotherapy was restarted. Ipilimumab was not restarted to reduce the risk of recurrence of his severe immune-mediated side effects. Although the transaminitis and colitis did not recur on nivolumab monotherapy, the patient did go on to develop dramatic poliosis (hair whitening) and eyelashes, followed by immune-mediated adrenal insufficiency. The latter presented as abdominal pain, dizziness and fatigue associated with hypotension. This was treated with hydrocortisone supplementation.

Interval imaging at 6 and 12 months follow-up showed complete resolution of the brain metastases, and the immunotherapy was discontinued after a total of a year and a half of therapy given the complete response on his radiologic studies. The patient is currently 2 years from the initial presentation and is disease-free and off all immunotherapy.

Discussion

- More than one-third of patients diagnosed with metastatic melanoma have brain metastases at the time of diagnosis, portending a poor prognosis with a median survival of 4 months. Though surgical resection and stereotactic radiation are useful for solitary metastases, effective well-tolerated treatments are limited in the setting of multiple brain metastases.[1]

- Immune checkpoint inhibitors include the anti-CTLA-4 antibody, ipilimumab, and the anti-PD-1 antibodies nivolumab and pembrolizumab, augment host immune responses to tumors by abrogating T-cell inactivation.[2]

- This form of immune therapy results in frequent immune-mediated adverse events (IRAEs), most often affecting the skin, gastrointestinal tract, liver, endocrine glands, and lungs.[3] Although anti-PD-1 and anti-CTLA-4 agents share similar toxicity profiles, ipilimumab has a greater frequency of grade 3–4 side effects. In comparison, the toxicities associated with anti-PD-1 therapy are often better tolerated. The combination of ipilimumab and nivolumab has a greater efficacy than either agent alone. However, combination therapy is also associated with a particularly high rate of immune-mediated toxicity that often necessitates discontinuation of therapy. The CheckMate-067 trial reported grade 3–4 adverse events in 59% of patients receiving combination therapy compared to 21% in those receiving nivolumab monotherapy and 28% in the ipilimumab monotherapy groups.[3,4]

- Dermatological adverse events are the most frequent IRAEs seen for all checkpoint inhibitors and include maculopapular rash, pruritus, and vitiligo. The skin is also usually the first organ to be affected by IRAEs, typically in the first 4–6 weeks after starting treatment. Though dermatological side effects are common, they tend to be grade 1–2 severity and easily manageable, typically not requiring discontinuation of therapy. On the positive side, these reactions, primarily rash and vitiligo, have also been associated with better survival outcomes.[5]

- Gastrointestinal side effects are the next most commonly seen adverse reactions and include diarrhea and colitis, both of which are seen more frequently in regimens that include ipilimumab.[6] About 5%–10% of patients develop an endocrine abnormality affecting the pituitary, thyroid, or adrenal gland. These toxicities are frequently permanent.[3] Hepatic function is routinely monitored during treatment due to the risk of hepatotoxicity, presenting as elevated AST/ALT and bilirubin, again seen more often with combination therapy.[3]

- Most of these immune-mediated effects are reversible and can be managed with a treatment break and a tapering course of corticosteroids. Less frequently, anti-TNF therapy with agents such as infliximab or anti-integrin therapies such as vedolizumab are used for steroid-refractory immune toxicity.[3]

- Combination therapy with nivolumab and ipilimumab has been found to be more efficacious for melanoma metastatic to the brain than treatment with either therapy alone.[2] With regard to *BRAF*-mutant melanoma, although there are no direct comparison studies, combination therapy with nivolumab and ipilimumab suggests comparable efficacy with increased durable response compared to combination MEK/BRAF-targeted therapy. Therefore, combination immunotherapy should be considered first-line for melanoma patients with brain metastases.[2,7]

- In a retrospective, pooled study examining efficacy and safety outcomes in patients who discontinued combination immunotherapy due to adverse events it was found that approximately 40% of patients discontinued therapy. It is notable, however, that efficacy outcomes were similar in both groups, suggesting that treatment discontinuation due to toxicity may not negatively affect the treatment outcomes.[4]

Teaching Pearls

- Immune checkpoint inhibitors, anti-CTLA-4 and anti-PD-1, are commonly associated with immune-mediated adverse effects, which can affect almost any organ in the body.
- Although the combination of these therapies appears to be more effective in specific subgroups of patients with metastatic melanoma, including those with CNS metastases, this is associated with significantly increased toxicity that often necessitates drug discontinuation. Fortunately, this does not appear to affect efficacy outcomes from these drugs.

References

1. Davies M, Liu P, McIntyre S, et al. Prognostic factors for survival in melanoma patients with brain metastases. *Cancer.* 2011; 117(8): 1687–1696.
2. Larkin J, Chiarion-Sileni V, Gonzalez R, et al. Combined nivolumab and ipilimumab or monotherapy in untreated melanoma. *New Eng J Med.* 2015; 373: 23–34.
3. Sosa A, Cadena EL, Olive CS, et al. Clinical assessment of immune-related adverse events. *Ther Adv Med Oncol.* 2018; 10: 1–11.
4. Shadendorf D, Wolchok JD, Hodi FS, et al. Efficacy and safety outcomes in patients with advanced melanoma who discontinued treatment with nivolumab and ipilimumab because of adverse events: a pooled analysis of randomized phase II and III trials. *J Clin Oncol.* 2017; 35(34): 3807–3814.
5. Rzepecki A, Cheng H, McLellan BN. Cutaneous toxicity as a predictive biomarker for clinical outcome in patients receiving anticancer therapy. *J Am Acad Dermatol.* 2018; 79(3): 545–555.
6. Michot, JM, Bigenwald C, Champiat S, et al. Immune-related adverse events with immune checkpoint blockade: a comprehensive review. *Eur J Cancer.* 2016; 54: 139–148.
7. Tawbi H, Boutros C, Kok D, et al. New era in management of melanoma brain metastases. *Am Soc Clin Oncol Educ Book.* 2018; 38: 741–750.

Case 1.5

Authors: Marguerite Sullivan, MD, Sara Al Janahi MD, MSc, Iman Fatima Khan, MS, MPH, and Adam Lerner, MD.

Reason for Presentation: Stage IV melanoma presenting as epidermotropic cutaneous melanoma metastases successfully treated with combination targeted therapy.

Chief Complaint: Multiple new bumps on the body.

History of Present Illness: A patient presented to the clinic with a 6-month history of multiple new enlarging bumps that started on the left thigh and gradually spread to the upper extremity, trunk, and neck. The lesions were intensely pruritic. Of note, the patient's history was significant for stage III melanoma of the left cheek 3 years prior to this presentation.

Review of Systems: No pertinent positives.

Medical/Surgical History: Stage III malignant melanoma (amelanotic) of the left cheek treated with WLE, CLND, and radiation to the nodal basin.

Medications: None.

Family History: No pertinent positives.

Social History: Nil relevant.

Physical Examination: A large surgical scar on the left cheek extending down to the left side of the neck, with no evidence of pigmentation or nodularity within the scar; Neck/chest/back/abdomen, upper extremities, and lower extremities with scattered 4–8 mm skin-colored to reddish-brown, firm, dermal papules that were non-tender (see Figure 1.5.1); Lymph nodes: No palpable cervical, axillary, or inguinal lymph nodes.

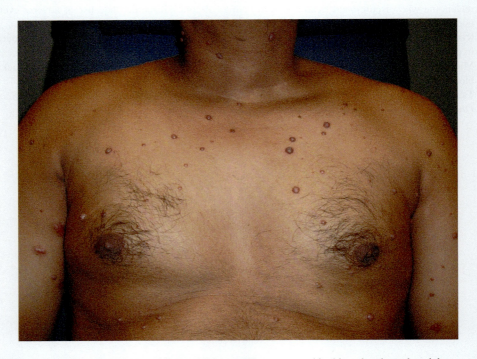

FIGURE 1.5.1 Pre-systemic therapy – widespread, innumerable, monomorphic skin-colored papulonodules.

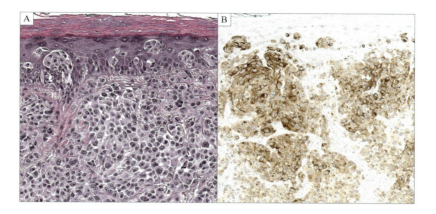

FIGURE 1.5.2 Punch biopsy of a papule on the left outer thigh: (A) H&E, high power and (B) MART-1 immunostain.

Pathology: Punch biopsy of a papule on the left outer thigh (see Figure 1.5.2): (A) Epidermis showed nests and single atypical melanocytes with pagetoid spread and similar melanocytes with plasmacytoid (arrow) and binucleate (arrowhead) morphology in the dermis (H&E, 200×). (B) Tumor cells were positive with immunoperoxidase staining for Mart-1 (200×) consistent with malignant melanoma.

Investigations

- **Brain MRI:** No evidence of metastases.
- **Whole-body PET-CT:** Multiple cutaneous hypermetabolic 3–9 mm lesions; no other metastases elsewhere.

Final Diagnosis: Stage IV malignant melanoma with multiple epidermotropic cutaneous metastases.

Management and Disease Course

At the time of diagnosis for this patient, the FDA had recently approved the anti-CTLA-4 drug, ipilimumab, for the treatment of metastatic melanoma. The patient was started on the drug and completed a 12-week course. While on therapy, however, the skin lesions continued to increase in size and number, and disease progression was confirmed by an interval PET-CT scan. During the patient's clinical progression on ipilimumab therapy, the FDA also approved the use of combination targeted therapy with BRAF and MEK inhibitors for the treatment of patients with BRAF-mutant metastatic melanoma. Genetic testing on one of the cutaneous metastases confirmed that the patient's melanoma carried the *V600E* mutation. Treatment was then switched from ipilimumab to dabrafenib and trametinib combination therapy. Within 2 weeks, the cutaneous lesions changed from being skin-colored to dark brown, pigmented papules (see Figure 1.5.3). Soon after, the lesions were noted to shrink significantly, and within 6 months all the lesions were either flat or completely resolved. The response was maintained and the patient continued this therapy without evidence of new lesions for the following 4 years.

While on targeted therapy, the patient developed hyperglycemia and uveitis, which were attributed to his therapy. This was treated with metformin and steroid eye drops, respectively, without any interruption in the patient's regimen. The patient was able to continue life in the usual way without any further symptoms.

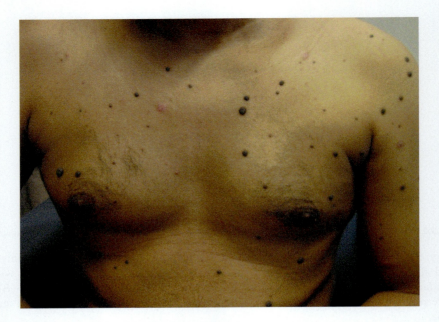

FIGURE 1.5.3   Post-targeted therapy – rapid pigmentation of the papulonodules.

Discussion

- While cutaneous metastases of melanoma typically involve the dermis and subcutaneous fat, epidermotropic metastatic melanoma, a rare presentation, shows tropism and involvement of the epidermis and superficial dermis. This can make these lesions difficult to distinguish from a primary melanoma on a skin biopsy and lead to missing the diagnosis of stage IV disease on histopathology alone. Clinicopathological correlation can interpret the occurrence of multiple synchronous lesions of melanoma as being lesions of epidermotropic cutaneous melanoma metastases. This can alert the physician to the much worse prognosis for the patient that is associated with stage IV disease and help direct management appropriately.[1]

- The MAPK pathway leads to cellular proliferation and survival. BRAF is a protein kinase that is an integral component of this pathway. It is mutated in ~50% of melanomas due to a point mutation at amino acid residue 600, most commonly with glutamic acid replacing the wild-type valine residue. This leads to constitutive activation of the MAPK pathway and cellular proliferation.[2] BRAF inhibitors such as vemurafenib and dabrafenib show antitumor activity in melanoma that is positive for the *BRAF* mutation.

- Common adverse effects seen with BRAF inhibitors include arthralgia, rash, fatigue, alopecia, nausea, and diarrhea. Toxicities specific to dabrafenib include fevers and hyperglycemia, while those specific to vemurafenib include prolongation of QT interval, peripheral facial palsy, and reduced creatinine clearance.[2,3] The development of single or multiple SCCs, typically of the keratoacanthoma type, occurs in 15%–25% of patients treated with BRAF inhibitors. This phenomenon is attributed to paradoxical activation of the MAPK pathway in precancerous keratinocytes displaying wild-type *BRAF* that harbor an upstream activating mutation in H-Ras.[4]

- MEK is another protein kinase that functions downstream from BRAF in the MAPK pathway. MEK inhibitors, including trametinib, binimetinib, and cobimetinib, have shown improved survival when compared to chemotherapy in the treatment of *BRAF*-mutated melanoma. Common toxicities of MEK inhibitors include diarrhea, edema, rash, and, less commonly, reversibly decreased cardiac ejection fraction and retinopathy.[5]

- BRAF inhibitors show significant response rates of >50% and improved overall and progression-free survival in patients with advanced *BRAF*-mutated melanoma. Despite their efficacy, the major disadvantage with these medications is the temporary nature of the response, with the inevitable development of drug resistance and disease relapse in a median duration of 6–7 months.[2–6] The causes of resistance are myriad and include both genetic and epigenetic alterations in the tumor that ultimately lead to reactivation of the MAPK pathway.

- The addition of a MEK inhibitor to a BRAF inhibitor has the theoretical capability of causing greater efficacy by causing dual inhibition of the MAPK pathway. By blocking the MAPK pathway downstream of BRAF, MEK inhibitors also reduce some of the side effects from BRAF inhibitors that are due to paradoxical activation of MAPK in wild-type BRAF cells. These hypotheses were borne true in a randomized control trial which demonstrated greater efficacy and a more durable response of combination targeted therapy versus BRAF inhibitor monotherapy in the treatment of advanced melanoma. As might have been expected, there was a lower incidence of keratoacanthoma-type SCC. Adverse effects from the combination targeted therapy include increased febrile syndromes with dabrafenib and trametinib and increased diarrhea, nausea, rash, and liver abnormalities with vemurafenib and cobimetinib.[5–8]

- While treatment with BRAF and MEK inhibitors is a valuable form of therapy for many patients with *BRAF*-mutant melanoma, it should be noted that the 5-year OS for dabrafenib and trametinib-treated patients is 34%, and the disease-free survival rate is 19%. These results do not compare favorably with combination immune checkpoint therapy (ipilimumab and nivolumab) where the 5-year OS rate is 60% in *BRAF*-mutant melanoma patients, with a corresponding disease-free survival rate of 38%. Given this recent long-term follow-up data, many oncologists would consider combined immune checkpoint inhibitors as front-line therapy for BRAF-mutated melanoma patients.[7,9]

Teaching Pearls

- BRAF and MEK inhibitors given in combination versus as monotherapy is a standard of care in *BRAF*-mutated melanomas. The combination therapy has greater efficacy and durability of response.

- Toxicities, including diarrhea and rash, are common with BRAF/MEK inhibitor therapy. However, the combination negates the paradoxical activation of wild-type BRAF, leading to a reduced risk of developing cutaneous SCCs.

References

1. Kim H, So B, Yo MG, et al. Epidermotropic metastatic melanoma clinically resembling agminated spitz nevi. *Ann Dermatol*. 2015; 26(5): 628–631.
2. Hauschild A, Grob J, Demidov L, et al. Dabrafenib in BRAF-mutated metastatic melanoma: a multi-center, open-label, phase 3 randomised controlled trial. *Lancet*. 2012; 380: 358.
3. Chapman P, Hauschild A, Robert C, et al. Improved survival with vemurafenib in melanoma with BRAF V600E mutation. *N Engl J Med*. 2011; 264: 2507.
4. Su F, Viros A, Milagre C, et al. RAS mutations in cutaneous squamous-cell carcinomas in patients treated with BRAF inhibitors. *N Engl J Med*. 2012; 366(3): 207–215.
5. Hu-Lieskovan S, Robert L, Moreno BH, et al. Combining targeted therapy with immunotherapy in BRAF-mutant melanoma: promise and challenges. *J Clin Oncol*. 2014; 32(21): 2248–2254. doi:10.1200/JCO.2013.52.1377.
6. Luke J, Flaherty K, Ribas A, et al. Targeted agents and immunotherapies: optimizing outcomes in melanoma. *Nat Rev Clin Oncol*. 2018; 14(8): 463–482.
7. Robert C, Grob J, Stroyakovskiy D, et al. Five-year outcomes with dabrafenib plus trametinib in metastatic melanoma. *N Engl J Med*. 2019; 381(7): 626–636.
8. Ascierto P, McArthur G. Cobimetinib combined with vemurafenib in advanced BRAF(V600)-mutant melanoma (coBRIM): updated efficacy results from a randomized, double-blind, phase 3 trial. *Lancet Oncol*. 2016; 17(9): 1248–1260.
9. Larkin J, Chiarion-Sileni V, Gonzalez R, et al. Five-year survival with combined nivolumab and ipilimumab in advanced melanoma. *N Engl J Med*. 2019; 381(16): 1535–1546.

Case 1.6

Authors: Bilal Fawaz, MD, Sarah Ann Kam, MD, Sara Al Janahi MD, MSc, Iman Fatima Khan, MS, MPH, and Debjani Sahni, MD.

Reason for Presentation: Treatment of incompletely excised melanoma in situ with imiquimod in a patient with multiple comorbidities.

History of Present Illness: An elderly patient presented with a 6-month history of a slowly growing, pink papule overlying an eczematous plaque on the right mid-abdomen. The lesion occasionally bled but was otherwise asymptomatic.

Review of Systems: No pertinent positives.

Medical/Surgical History: Multiple comorbidities including prior non-melanoma skin cancers; head and neck cancers, atrial fibrillation, and severe chronic obstructive pulmonary disease requiring home oxygen.

Medications: Warfarin, prednisone.

Family History: Melanoma.

Physical Examination: A frail patient in no acute distress, Fitzpatrick skin type I.

Abdomen: Right upper abdomen with coalescing pink, crusted papulonodules; no cervical, axillary, or inguinal lymphadenopathy.

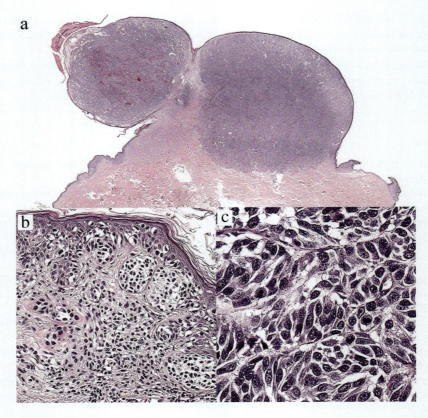

FIGURE 1.6.1 Incisional biopsy of the right upper abdomen papulonodule: (a) H&E, 10×; (b) H&E, 200×; and (c) H&E, 400×.

Pathology: Incisional biopsy of the right upper abdomen papulonodule (see Figure 1.6.1): (a) An exophytic nodular tumor (H&E, 10×). (b) Higher power revealing atypical melanocytes in the epidermis and dermis with pagetoid spread (H&E, 200×). (c) The dermal component exhibits mitotic activity (H&E, 400×). Consistent with malignant melanoma, nodular type.

Investigations

- **CT chest, abdomen, pelvis:** No evidence of metastasis.

Final Diagnosis: Amelanotic malignant melanoma on the abdomen.

Management and Disease Course: According to the NCCN guidelines for a pathological stage T4aNxMx melanoma, a WLE with an SLNB was considered. However, given the patient's comorbidities and risk of undergoing a general anesthetic, an SLNB was deferred. At the time of presentation of this patient, adjuvant therapy for melanoma had not yet been approved. The risk of undergoing an SLNB procedure significantly outweighed the benefit of prognostic information gained from an SLNB. A WLE was, therefore, performed under local anesthesia after a CT chest, abdomen, and pelvis confirmed no evidence of metastasis.

Following the WLE, the excision margins were found to be positive for invasive melanoma, requiring a second WLE. This also resulted in positive margins. A third WLE with 1 cm margins was recommended, and this time the margins were positive for melanoma in situ (MMis), with no evidence of an invasive component. The amelanotic nature of this melanoma made it challenging to assess clinical margins even with scouting biopsies. What was thought to be an eczematous rash around the original pink melanoma papule turned out to be part of the melanoma and its peripheral MMis (see Figure 1.6.2).

Following three consecutive WLEs on the abdomen, it became increasingly difficult to perform further WLE under local anesthesia. As a result, the cutaneous oncology tumor board panel recommended the use of imiquimod 5 days a week for 12 weeks applying this to a 2 cm margin around the WLE scar. After 4 weeks of therapy, imiquimod was held for 2 weeks as the patient experienced a

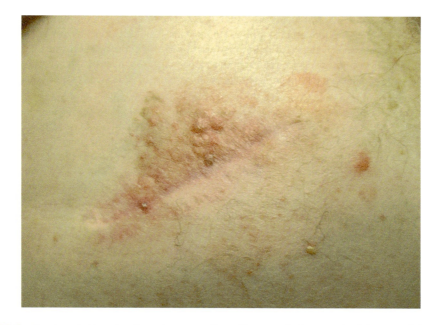

FIGURE 1.6.2 Agminated skin-colored papules surrounding a linear surgical scar on the right upper abdomen.

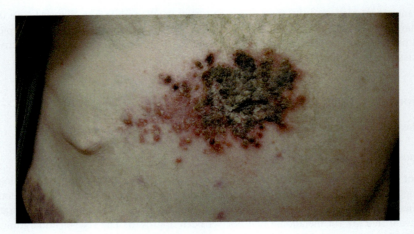

FIGURE 1.6.3 Grouped erythematous papulopustules coalescing around the surgical scar with overlying thick crust on the right upper abdomen.

robust inflammatory reaction on the abdomen with severe crusting (see Figure 1.6.3). On restarting application of imiquimod, it was decreased to 3 days a week. The patient experienced a severe inflammatory response even on this regimen, and so therapy had to be decreased to 1 day per week until completion of a total of 12 weeks of therapy. At the end of the treatment course, there was no evidence of residual lesions clinically, and subsequent scouting biopsies were all negative for melanoma and MMis at the 16-month follow-up visit.

Discussion

- Topical imiquimod is a viable treatment option for MMis in patients who are not good surgical candidates, with the greatest use in lentigo maligna (LM) subtype.[1–5] Imiquimod is a toll-like receptor 7 (TLR-7) agonist that stimulates the innate and acquired immune responses, leading to an antitumoral inflammatory state while inhibiting regulatory feedback mechanisms. Specifically, imiquimod acts on the nuclear factor κB signaling pathway to increase levels of interferon α and β as well as TNF-α.[1] Imiquimod also inhibits angiogenesis and activates the caspase pathway to induce cell apoptosis.[1,2] Evidence of imiquimod use for MMis in the neoadjuvant setting is limited, but it has been increasingly reported both as a primary treatment modality in non-surgical candidates and as adjuvant treatment in patients with residual in situ disease following surgery.[1–5]

- A systematic literature review concluded that the application of imiquimod 5 days a week for 12 weeks (on average >60 applications) has superior efficacy in treating MMis, with a clearance rate of 76.2%–78.3%.[1] The data came from retrospective chart reviews and open-label interventional studies. A large retrospective chart review study by Pandit et al. included 22 post-surgical patients with persistent positive margins for MMis after excision of the original melanoma or MMis.[3] Patients were treated with imiquimod 3–5 times per week for up to 12 weeks. After an average follow-up period of 2 years, 20/22 (95%) of patients demonstrated resolution of the residual disease, confirmed clinically and by diagnostic tissue biopsy. Of the 22 patients, one was lost to follow-up and one patient did not respond (5%). There were no reports of disease recurrence.[3]

- It is worth noting that treating a 2 cm margin of normal skin around the surgical scar is recommended, and that therapy should be adjusted according to the patient's reaction to imiquimod.[3] If daily use results in minimal inflammation, adding a daily topical retinoid (e.g., tretinoin 0.1% or tazarotene 0.1% cream/gel) is recommended. If the inflammatory response remains limited, then the application can be escalated to twice daily.[3] The main treatment goal is to achieve sustained inflammation for >12 weeks. On the other hand, if patients develop an exuberant inflammatory reaction with daily use, a 2-week break is advised followed by restarting treatment at a lower application frequency (e.g., three times weekly).[3] The patients in Pandit et al.'s protocol were followed every 2–4 weeks to assess treatment response and make necessary adjustments.[3]

- In another retrospective study, 63 cases of LM were treated with topical imiquimod either as primary therapy (22/63 or 34.9%) or adjuvant therapy of incompletely excised surgical margins (41/63; 65.1%).[4] After a mean treatment duration of 11.7 weeks and a mean follow-up time of 42.1 months, clinical clearance was achieved in 72.7% of primary tumors and 94.4% of tumors in the adjuvant group.[4] However, only 25.9% of the cases underwent post-treatment scouting biopsies to confirm histological clearance. The authors concluded that imiquimod may be used as either primary or adjuvant therapy of MMis in patients who are not good surgical candidates.[4]

- Topical imiquimod has a favorable side effect profile compared to surgery. The most common side effects are erythema and pain, and in more severe cases, vesicular inflammation with scabbing and crusting followed by post-inflammatory hyper/hypopigmentation. Imiquimod has the capability of being absorbed through the skin which can cause unintended systemic side effects such as cytokine-release syndrome. This includes fever, malaise, fatigue, and headaches. In the study by Pandit et al., one patient even developed depression while applying imiquimod, which improved after stopping the drug. The manufacturer's recommendation is to apply imiquimod to no more than a 25 cm^2 area of the skin. Adverse effects generally resolve upon discontinuation of therapy, following which the drug can be restarted at a lower frequency.[4]

- Despite the promising efficacy of imiquimod, surgical excision continues to be the standard of care for MMis.[2] Long-term, randomized controlled trials (RCTs) are still needed to compare the two treatment modalities. Additionally, published studies on imiquimod are of limited patient numbers in few institutions and they vary considerably in their methodology (frequency/duration of application, outcome assessment), hence limiting their generalizability.[1–5] Treatment efficacy in the aforementioned studies was determined by a variety of methods, including clinical evaluation alone, scouting biopsies, and re-excisions with 1 mm margins.[3–5] Due to study heterogeneity and the lack of RCTs, imiquimod remains a category 2B recommendation according to the NCCN guidelines (i.e., recommendation based upon lower-level evidence).[2] Together with close clinical monitoring, imiquimod may be a reasonable treatment option for MMis in patients who wish to avoid surgery or have multiple comorbidities that precludes them from extensive surgery.[2]

Teaching Pearls

- Surgery remains the first-line treatment for MMis. However, topical imiquimod may be used as a primary treatment modality for MMis in non-surgical candidates, or as adjuvant treatment in patients with residual in situ disease following initial surgical resection.
- Treatment should be adjusted based on the patient's reaction to imiquimod. The goal should be >60 applications of imiquimod, applied once a day, at least 3–5 times a week, for 12 weeks, and application should include a 2 cm margin of skin surrounding the lesion or surgical scar.

References

1. Mora AN, Karia PS, Nguyen BM. A quantitative systematic review of the efficacy of imiquimod monotherapy for lentigo maligna and an analysis of factors that affect tumor clearance. *J Am Acad Dermatol.* 2015; 73(2): 205–212. doi:10.1016/j.jaad.2015.05.022.
2. Swetter SM, Tsao H, Bichakjian CK, et al. Guidelines of care for the management of primary cutaneous melanoma. *J Am Acad Dermatol.* 2019; 80(1): 208–250. doi:10.1016/j.jaad.2018.08.055.
3. Pandit AS, Geiger EJ, Ariyan S, et al. Using topical imiquimod for the management of positive in situ margins after melanoma resection. *Cancer Med.* 2015; 4(4): 507–512. doi:10.1002/cam4.402.
4. Swetter SM, Chen FW, Kim DD, et al. Imiquimod 5% cream as primary or adjuvant therapy for melanoma in situ, lentigo maligna type. *J Am Acad Dermatol.* 2015; 72(6): 1047–1053. doi:10.1016/j.jaad.2015.02.008.
5. Tsay C, Kim S, Norwich-Cavanaugh A, et al. An algorithm for the management of residual head and neck melanoma in situ using topical imiquimod: a pilot study. *Ann Plast Surg.* 2019; 82(4S Suppl 3): S199–S201. doi:10.1097/SAP.0000000000001840.

Case 1.7

Authors: Sarah Kam, MD, Tatchai Ruangrattanatavorn, MD, MSc, Elizabeth T. Rotrosen, AB, and Teviah E. Sachs, MD, MPH.

Reason for Presentation: Function-sparing management approach for an elderly patient with acral melanoma.

Chief Complaint: Lesion on the right foot.

History of Present Illness: An octogenarian presented for evaluation of a painful, enlarging ulcerated growth on the plantar surface of the right foot. There was a 10-year history of a painless, dark lesion in the same area. In the year prior to presentation, the lesion became pruritic and painful and developed ulceration.

Review of Systems: No pertinent positives.

Medical/Surgical History: Hypertension.

Medications: None.

Family History: No family history of skin cancer.

Social History: Recently emigrated from Haiti.

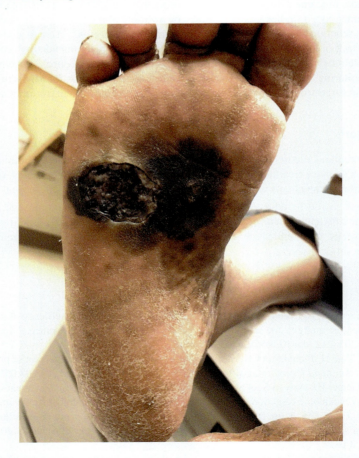

FIGURE 1.7.1   Irregular black-brown ulcer with surrounding irregularly pigmented macules and patches on the right plantar foot.

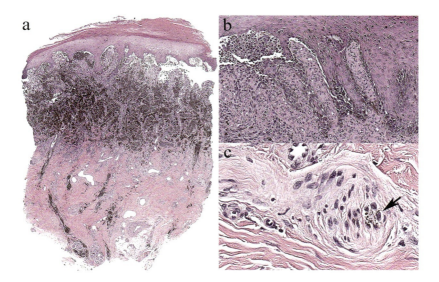

FIGURE 1.7.2   Punch biopsy of the large pigmented patch on the right plantar foot: (a) H&E, 10×; (b) H&E, 100×; and (c) H&E, 200×.

Physical Examination: Plantar surface of the right foot (see Figure 1.7.1): 7.0 × 5.0 cm brown-black oval patch with irregular borders. Within this patch, a 3.0 × 2.5 cm area of ulceration was present, in addition to light brown oval macules coalescing into a larger patch; no palpable inguinal, axillary, or cervical lymphadenopathy.

Pathology: Punch biopsy of the right plantar foot (see Figure 1.7.2): (a) Acral skin with deeply invading pigmented tumor (H&E, 10×). (b) Lentiginous proliferation of dyscohesive melanocytes with marked pagetoid scatter (H&E, 100×). (c) Pigmented spindle cells within a nerve twig consistent with intraneural invasion (H&E, 200×). Consistent with malignant melanoma, acral lentiginous type.

Pre-Operative Diagnosis: Melanoma at least stage IIb (T3bNxMx).

Management and Disease Course

The patient had a good functional status and enjoyed being independently mobile. In fact, this latter point was very important to her and something she did not want to sacrifice. A staging whole-body PET-CT and brain MRI were obtained, which revealed regional lymphadenopathy of the right inguinal region suspicious for malignancy. The NCCN guidelines recommend a biopsy of suspicious nodal disease and resection of the primary melanoma with 2 cm margins. An ultrasound-guided needle biopsy of the suspicious inguinal node was undertaken which was negative for malignancy. The lymphadenopathy was deemed to be reactive, secondary to the chronic inflammation from tumor ulceration; however, microscopic disease could not be excluded. The patient was recommended further evaluation of the nodal status with an SLNB, but deferred this due to the associated morbidity with this procedure. Performing a 2 cm margin WLE of the primary melanoma would result in the patient losing the fifth toe with associated significant issues post-operatively with mobility and function. Given this patient's stage in life and strong personal desire to maintain quality of life, a function-sparing surgical approach was suggested by the cutaneous oncology tumor board. A 2 cm margin was recommended around the biopsy-proven invasive component of the tumor, whereas a 0.5 cm margin was advised around the lighter brown periphery of the tumor which had shown only in situ disease on biopsy. The patient agreed to this approach and tolerated the function-sparing WLE well without significant impact to mobility and quality of life.

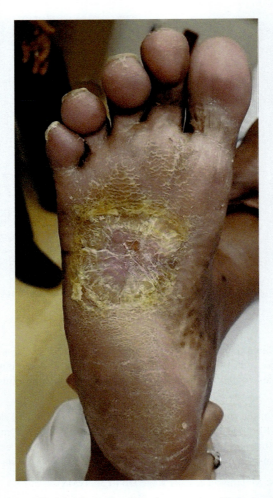

FIGURE 1.7.3 Well-healed scar on the right plantar foot following surgery and imiquimod therapy.

Five months following surgery, suspicious pigmentation was noted at the surgical margin. Biopsy was recommended by the team but declined by the patient, despite being warned that this may be a sign of cancer recurrence. With the presumptive diagnosis being recurrence of the MMis component at the surgical margin, the patient was treated with imiquimod 5% cream, 5 days a week for 12 weeks. This resulted in complete clinical resolution of the pigmentation (see Figure 1.7.3). Inguinal lymph nodes were monitored with regular clinical examination and ultrasound scan at 3–4 months intervals for the next 1 year. No adenopathy was found and the patient remains free of recurrence 3 years after her initial presentation.

Discussion

- As healthcare providers, our duty is to enable patients to make informed decisions that align with their personal expectations of healthcare and quality of life goals. In this case, the patient's main wish was to remain functionally independent, fully ambulatory, and minimize chronic pain. A 2 cm margin around the entire acral melanoma would have led to the loss of the right fifth toe with consequent prolonged wound healing, limited mobility, and some loss of function of the right foot. A function-sparing limited WLE was, therefore, undertaken instead. Given the absence of macroscopic nodal disease on the imaging scans, the patient did not wish to undergo the potential morbidity from an SLNB to check for microscopic disease, particularly as her presentation predated the approval of adjuvant systemic therapy in melanoma. Instead, close post-operative monitoring of the resection bed and the associated lymph node basins (with imaging) was advised.

- Surgery remains the gold standard for the treatment of resectable melanomas. WLE is most commonly employed, with variable margins determined by the depth of melanoma invasion.[1] The NCCN guidelines recommend 0.5–1.0 cm for MMis, 1.0 cm for melanomas ≤1.0 mm thick, 1–2 cm for melanoma thickness of 1.01–2 mm, 2 cm margins for melanoma thickness of 2.01–4 mm, and 2 cm margins for melanomas >4 mm thick.[1]

- Mohs micrographic surgery (MMS) has gained attention more recently as another viable surgical option due to the growing body of evidence demonstrating comparable outcomes to WLE.[1-3] MMS is advantageous due to its tissue-sparing nature and optimal margin control as 100% of the surgical margin is evaluated intra-operatively. This is particularly important in larger melanomas or in those occurring on cosmetically or functionally sensitive areas such as the face or acral surfaces.[1-3] The main disadvantage of MMS is the difficulty in interpreting melanocytic lesions on frozen sections when compared to permanent paraffin-embedded sections, especially on chronically sun-damaged skin.[2,3] However, the addition of MART-1 staining to MMS has dramatically improved the surgeon's intra-operative ability to evaluate melanoma specimens.[2] Several studies have since revealed either comparable or superior outcomes of MMS vs. WLE.[3-5] A recent retrospective cohort study evaluating 2,114 in situ and invasive melanomas revealed a local recurrence rate of 0.59% and a disease-specific survival of 98.53% after a mean follow-up time of 3.7 years.[2] Other studies comparing outcomes in both surgical modalities demonstrated no statistical difference in recurrence rates (5.7% in WLE group vs. 1.8% in MMS group, $P = 0.07$), five-year OS (94% in WLE group vs. 92% in MMS group, $P = 0.28$), and melanoma-specific mortality (6.1 years in WLE group vs. 6.5 years in MMS group, $P = 0.77$).[3] While surgical excision with paraffin-embedded sections continues to be the gold standard for evaluating atypical melanocytic lesions, MMS appears to be at least equally efficacious in the treatment of melanoma.[3-5] The experience of the Mohs surgeon in dealing with atypical pigmented lesions also plays a role in treatment success. Randomized, prospective studies are needed to determine which is the superior surgical modality in this setting. Our patient was offered MMS for the acral melanoma but declined as it would involve managing a large open wound for a week between the MMS and reconstructive surgery.

- Non-surgical options may be considered for less invasive disease in frail patients, those who decline surgery, or those whose lesions are in cosmetically or functionally sensitive areas. Most notably, imiquimod is a well-tolerated treatment for primary or residual MIS, with clearance rates of 76.2%–78.3% if applied >60 times (5 days a week for 12 weeks on average).[6] At our institution, we recommend the protocol from Pandit and colleagues at Yale, which consists of imiquimod 5% cream five times a week for at least 12 weeks.[7] The frequency and duration of application is adjusted to limit toxicity and maximize effect (discussed in detail in Case 1.6). The protocol has demonstrated a clearance rate of 95% after a mean follow-up period of 24 months.[7] Although our patient declined a post-imiquimod treatment biopsy to confirm disease clearance, the pigmentation from the presumed melanoma recurrence cleared completely using this protocol and has not recurred since.

Teaching Pearls

- Surgical resection remains the first-line treatment for melanoma. MMS has gained attention recently, especially for the LM subtype.
- In elderly or frail patients, surgical morbidity should be weighed against its benefits, and the patient's personal goals of care and quality of life must be taken into consideration when deciding on the treatment plan.
- Imiquimod is an appropriate and effective treatment option for residual MMis in non-surgical candidates.

References

1. Beaulieu D, Fathi R, Srivastava D, et al. Current perspectives on Mohs micrographic surgery for melanoma. *Clin Cosmet Investig Dermatol.* 2018; 11: 309–320. doi:10.2147/CCID.S137513.
2. Valentín-Nogueras SM, Brodland DG, Zitelli JA, et al. Mohs micrographic surgery using Mart-1 immunostains in the treatment of invasive melanoma and melanoma in situ. *Dermatol Surg.* 2016; 42(6): 733–744.
3. Nosrati A, Berliner JG, Goel S, et al. Outcomes of melanoma in situ treated with Mohs micrographic surgery compared with wide local excision. *JAMA Dermatol.* 2017; 153(5): 436–441. doi:10.1001/jamadermatol.2016.6138.
4. Trofymenko O, Bordeaux JS, Zeitouni NC. Melanoma of the face and Mohs micrographic surgery: nationwide mortality data analysis. *Dermatol Surg.* 2018; 44(4): 481–492.
5. Ellison PM, Zitelli JA, Brodland DG. Mohs micrographic surgery for melanoma: a prospective multicenter study. *J Am Acad Dermatol.* 2019; 81(3): 767–774.
6. Mora AN, Karia PS, Nguyen BM. A quantitative systematic review of the efficacy of imiquimod monotherapy for lentigo maligna and an analysis of factors that affect tumor clearance. *J Am Acad Dermatol.* 2015; 73(2): 205–212.
7. Pandit AS, Geiger EJ, Ariyan S, et al. Using topical imiquimod for the management of positive in situ margins after melanoma resection. *Cancer Med.* 2015; 4(4): 507–512. doi:10.1002/cam4.402.

Case 1.8

Authors: Sarah Phillips, MD, Malathi Chittireddy, MD, MSc, Hannah E. Mumber, BS, and Michael R. Cassidy, MD.

Reason for Presentation: Management approach for primary dermal melanoma.

Chief Complaint: Bump on the right arm.

History of Present Illness: A middle-aged patient of Irish decent with a history of actinic keratoses and rosacea presented for evaluation of an enlarging asymptomatic bump on the right forearm. The lesion was present since childhood but had recently increased in size. The patient denied any personal history of skin cancer. They reported a normal colonoscopy 5 years prior to presentation, and a normal ophthalmology exam 2 years prior to presentation.

Review of Systems: No pertinent positives.

Medical/Surgical History: Rosacea; actinic damage.

Medications: Metronidazole 0.75% cream, 5-fluorouracil 5% cream.

Social: Nil relevant.

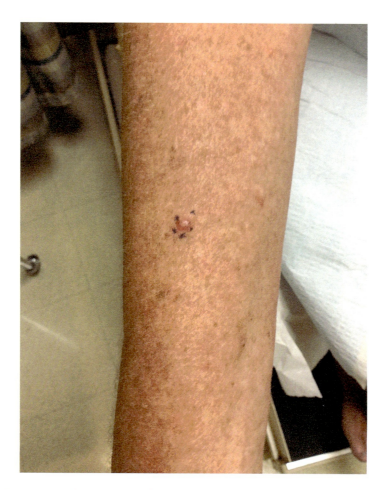

FIGURE 1.8.1 Pink papule on the right anterior forearm.

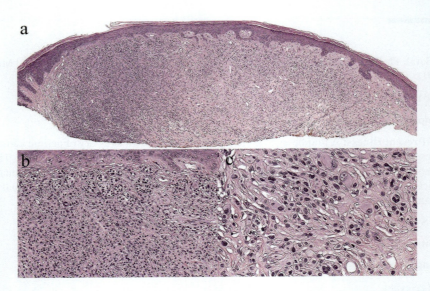

FIGURE 1.8.2 Shave biopsy of the papule on the right anterior forearm: (a) H&E, 40×; (b) H&E, 100×; and (c) H&E, 400×.

Family History: Positive for non-melanoma skin cancer.

Physical Examination: Right anterior forearm: With a pink dome-shaped papule with overlying telangiectasia (see Figure 1.8.1); Lymph nodes: No cervical, axillary, inguinal, or popliteal lymphadenopathy.

Pathology: Shave biopsy of the papule on the right anterior forearm (see Figure 1.8.2): (a) Diffuse dermal tumor (H&E, 40×). (b) Nests and sheets of melanocytes embedded in a fibrotic stroma with no junctional component (H&E, 100×). (c) Moderately to severely atypical epithelioid melanocytes with pleomorphic nuclei and prominent nucleoli (H&E, 400×). Consistent with dermal melanoma.

Investigations: A PET-CT scan of the whole body and brain MRI were normal.

Final Diagnosis: Primary dermal melanoma of the right forearm.

Management and Disease Course: Due to the absence of a junctional component on the skin biopsy, the differential diagnosis of this lesion included a metastatic melanoma from a distant primary versus a primary dermal melanoma. A thorough skin examination did not reveal any atypical lesions suspicious for a potential melanoma primary and imaging studies were normal. Given this, a diagnosis of primary dermal melanoma was made (at least T2aNxMx; stage IIA). According to the NCCN guidelines, WLE of the primary dermal melanoma and SLNB were performed. Final surgical margins were negative, and the right antecubital and axillary sentinel lymph nodes were negative. There was no evidence of local or distant recurrence at 5 years follow-up.

Discussion

- Primary dermal melanoma (PDM) is a rare entity that was first categorized in 2004 but was previously described in 2000 as a solitary melanoma confined to the dermal and/or subcutaneous tissue without evidence of a primary tumor elsewhere.[1–3] PDM is hypothesized to arise from a malignant transformation of non-epidermal melanocytes, or from a primary cutaneous melanoma with a regressed epidermal component.[3]
- PDM was originally distinguished from *metastatic melanoma with unknown primary site* and nodular melanoma by its superior survival rate. Distinguishing PDM from *metastatic melanoma with unknown primary site* is, however, difficult. To date, this distinction is based upon

ruling out any other primary cutaneous or visceral melanoma or any evidence of metastatic melanoma elsewhere.[2] Although the literature on PDM is limited, it does suggest a better prognosis of this entity in comparison to stage matched conventional cutaneous melanoma.

- Histologically, PDM is indistinguishable from a cutaneous metastasis of melanoma. Efforts to characterize PDM based on other clinical and histological features have proved challenging. Although more research is needed, one recent study suggested that there may be lower levels of p53, Ki-67, cyclin D1, and D2-40 in PDM relative to both malignant melanoma and primary nodular melanoma.[4] Another study suggested that a melanoma prognostic assay could be a promising test to help distinguish PDM from cutaneous metastatic melanoma.[5] There is also a suggestion that PDM may have lower rates of *BRAF V600E* mutations relative to other cutaneous melanomas.[6] At present, however, there is no reliable way to distinguish PDM from a cutaneous metastasis of melanoma via histopathologic or immunohistochemical features.

Teaching Pearls

- PDM is a rare presentation and a diagnosis of exclusion.
- They should be approached with full-body skin examination, including an eye examination, complete body imaging, and age-appropriate colonoscopy screening to rule out an underlying occult primary melanoma or metastatic melanoma.

References

1. Bowen GM, Chang AE, Lowe L, et al. Solitary melanoma confined to the dermal and/or subcutaneous tissue: evidence for revisiting the staging classification. *Arch Dermatol.* 2000; 136: 1397–1399.
2. Swetter SM, Ecker PM, Johnson D, et al. Primary dermal melanoma: a distinct subtype of melanoma. *Arch Dermatol.* 2004; 140(1): 99–103.
3. Sini G, Colombino M, Lissia A, et al. Primary dermal melanoma in a patient with a history of multiple malignancies: a case report with molecular characterization. *Case Rep Dermatol.* 2013; 5: 192–197. doi: 10.1159/000354032.
4. Cassarino DS, Cabral ES, Kartha RV, et al. Primary dermal melanoma: distinct immunohistochemical findings and clinical outcome compared with nodular and metastatic melanoma. *Arch Dermatol.* 2008; 144(1): 49–56.
5. Sidiropoulos M, Obregon R, Sholl LM, et al. Primary dermal melanoma: a unique subtype of melanoma to be distinguished from cutaneous metastatic melanoma: a clinical, histologic, and gene expression–profiling study. *J Am Acad Dermatol.* 2014; 71: 1083–1092.
6. Teow J, Chin O, Hanikeri M, et al. Primary dermal melanoma: a west Australian cohort. *ANZ J Surg.* 2015; 85(9): 664–667.

2

Squamous Cell Carcinoma

Ali Al-Haseni and Debjani Sahni

CONTENTS

Introduction

Cutaneous squamous cell carcinoma (cSCC) is the second-most common skin cancer, representing 20%–50% of all skin cancers.[1,2] It occurs due to malignant transformation of epidermal keratinocytes or its appendages. It is more common in fair-skinned individuals and tends to arise in chronically sun-exposed areas of the skin.[2] cSCC can arise de novo, but more commonly grows from a precursor lesion such as actinic keratosis (AK) or squamous cell carcinoma in situ (cSCCis). It is more aggressive than basal cell carcinoma (BCC) and can cause significant morbidity and mortality if it metastasizes (5-year survival is 26%–34% in cSCC with nodal metastasis).[1–3] Surgical treatment continues to be the modality of choice to achieve cure, with few other therapeutic options offering a comparable cure rate.

Although cSCC is the second most common skin cancer in fair-skinned individuals, it is the most common skin cancer in people of color. The incidence of cSCC has increased by 263% between 1976 and 2010, and it is predicted to continue to rise due to an aging world population and improved cancer screening. The exact incidence of cSCC in the United States (US) is difficult to calculate, as cSCC and BCC are not included in US cancer registries. Data from Europe and Australia show an incidence of 5–96 per 100,000 persons and 291–499 per 100,000 persons, respectively.[3] A national population data study from the US reported that roughly 600,000 patients were treated for cSCC in 2006.[2,4]

cSCC is characterized by the highest mutational burden of all solid cancers.[5] Multiple gene mutations have been observed in cSCC, with the most common mutation being *tumor protein 53* (*TP53*), enabling tumor cells to resist apoptosis. Other common mutations include *NOTCH1*, *Ras*, *cyclin-dependent kinase inhibitor 2A* (*CDKN2A*), and *epidermal growth factor receptor* (*EGFR*), among others, most of which occur due to UV radiation.[1,2]

The most important risk factors for the development of cSCC are chronic sun exposure, fair skin type, immune suppression (65–250 increased risk), and increased age (>60 years of age).[1,2] Other risk factors include male sex (3:1 ratio), prior radiation, tanning bed use, human papillomaviruses (HPV) 16 and 18 infections, certain radiosensitive genetic conditions (e.g., xeroderma pigmentosum), chronic wounds, chronic inflammation (e.g., discoid lupus), as well as environmental exposure to arsenic, polycyclic aromatic hydrocarbons (tar, pitch, and soot), nitrosamines, and alkylating agents. Lastly, certain cancer medications are associated with increased incidence of cSCC, specifically BRAF inhibitors such as vemurafenib.[1,2,6]

DOI: 10.1201/9780429026683-2

cSCC typically presents as a changing growth within an AK. Neoplastic change should be suspected if there is excessive hyperkeratosis, base induration, tenderness, or ulceration. De novo cSCC presents as an asymptomatic enlarging red papule or plaque with white scale. With time, these lesions tend to enlarge, ulcerate, or undergo central necrosis. The tumor arises in chronically sun-exposed areas in 90% of cases, with the head and neck being the most common sites in males, and the upper extremities followed by the head and neck in females. The risk of metastasis is relatively low and ranges from 3% to 5%, but once present, it is associated with a median survival of less than 2 years. The most common sites of metastasis are the regional lymph nodes, followed by the lungs, liver, brain, skin, and bones.[2]

cSCC is characterized by full-thickness keratinocytic atypia originating from the epidermis and infiltrating the dermis. Prominent keratinization and extracellular horn pearls can be seen. The cells are pleomorphic with high degrees of atypia and frequent mitoses. Many pathological variants of cSCC have been described, and this carries significance as certain variants have shown a higher risk of recurrence and metastasis. These high-risk variants include desmoplastic cSCC (characterized by an infiltrative growth pattern in combination with large amounts of stroma and narrow cords of cells), acantholytic cSCC (characterized by intratumoral glandular-like structures secondary to acantholysis), adenosquamous cSCC (characterized by the coexistence of malignant keratinocytes and atypical mucosecretory tubular structures), and metaplastic cSCC (characterized by sarcomatous changes).

The National Comprehensive Cancer Network (NCCN) divides cSCC into high- and low-risk cancers based on their propensity for recurrence or metastasis. High-risk factors are based on clinical and pathological factors. Clinical factors include tumor of any size in high-risk (H) areas (mask areas of the face, namely, central face, eyelids, eyebrow, periorbital, nose, lips, chin, mandible, pre/postauricular, temple, and ears; genitalia; hands and feet), tumors equal to or larger than 1 cm in medium-risk (M) areas (cheeks, forehead, scalp, neck, and pretibial region), tumors equal to or larger than 2 cm in low-risk (L) areas (trunk and extremities, excluding hands, nail, pretibial region, ankles, and feet). Other risk factors include tumors with poorly defined borders, recurrent tumors, tumors in immunosuppressed individuals at sites of prior radiation or chronic inflammation, or tumors that are rapidly growing or causing neurological symptoms. The high-risk histopathological factors include poor differentiation, depth over 6 mm, invasion beyond subcutaneous fat, perineural/lymphatic/vascular invasion, or certain histological growth patterns (acantholytic, adenosquamous, desmoplastic, or metaplastic subtypes).[7]

The overall prognosis and survival for the majority of patients with cSCC is excellent, with 5-year cure rates exceeding 90%.[2] Surgical excision with margin assessment is considered the first-line treatment to achieve complete cure.[2] The NCCN recommends excision with 4–6 mm margins along with post-operative margin assessment for low-risk cSCC, and excision with wider surgical margins or Mohs micrographic surgery for high-risk cSCC. The NCCN does not recommend specific defined margins for high-risk cSCCs, given the wide variety of factors constituting high-risk tumors. Instead, they recommend modifying the margins to adjust for specific patient and tumor factors.[7]

Radiation therapy (RT) is an alternative treatment option for non-surgical candidates. RT offers the advantage of treating subclinical extension through a field margin, and it can be used either as primary treatment or in the adjuvant setting.[2] It is typically reserved for older patients (>60 years old) due to concern for potential long-term sequelae (most importantly, radiation-induced malignancies). The recurrence rate is less than 7.9%.[8] Complications of radiation are divided into acute and late. Acute complications are usually encountered during or shortly after treatment and include erythema, moist desquamation, and fatigue. Late complications are encountered months to years after treatment and include skin dyspigmentation, hair loss, telangiectasias, and skin atrophy. Absolute contraindications to the use of radiation include previously radiated tumors that received the maximum radiation dose, as well as patients with radiation hypersensitivity syndromes (e.g., xeroderma pigmentosum). Relative contraindications include young age (<40 years old), lower limb (due to poor wound healing), connective tissue disease (such as scleroderma or lupus), peripheral vascular disease, and patients who are less able to cooperate (e.g., movement disorders or dementia).[11]

Systemic therapies are used mostly for metastatic cSCCs but are also considered for unresectable disease or when RT is not possible. In recent years, two classes of therapies have emerged for cSCC treatment: Targeted and immunologic therapies. The main targeted therapy is in the form of EGFR inhibitors (e.g., cetuximab). EGFR is expressed in more than 90% of cSCC and is responsible for cellular proliferation, survival, angiogenesis, and metastasis. In 2006, the FDA approved cetuximab for the treatment of locally advanced or metastatic mucosal SCC. Its use in cSCC is still off-label. The other form of systemic treatment currently approved for use in cSCC is checkpoint inhibitor immunotherapy, specifically the PD-1 inhibitor cemiplimab.[12]

References

1. Que SKT, Zwald FO, Schmults CD. Cutaneous squamous cell carcinoma: incidence, risk factors, diagnosis, and staging. *J Am Acad Dermatol*. 2018;78(2):237–247. doi:10.1016/j.jaad.2017.08.059.

2. Stratigos A, Garbe C, Lebbe C, et al. Diagnosis and treatment of invasive squamous cell carcinoma of the skin: European consensus-based interdisciplinary guideline. *Eur J Cancer*. 2015;51(14):1989–2007. doi:10.1016/j.ejca.2015.06.110.

3. Keena Que ST, Zwald FO, Schmults CD, et al. Cutaneous squamous cell carcinoma: management of advanced and high-stage tumors. *J Am Acad Dermatol*. 2018;78(2):249–261 doi:10.1016/j.jaad.2017.08.058.

4. Karia PS, Han J, Schmults CD. Cutaneous squamous cell carcinoma: estimated incidence of disease, nodal metastasis, and deaths from disease in the United States, 2012. *J Am Acad Dermatol*. 2013;68(6):957–966. doi:10.1016/j.jaad.2012.11.037.

5. Pickering CR, Zhou JH, Lee JJ, et al. Mutational landscape of aggressive cutaneous squamous cell carcinoma. *Clin Cancer Res*. 2014;20(24):6582–6592. doi:10.1158/1078-0432.CCR-14-1768.

6. Jaju PD, Ransohoff KJ, Tang JY, et al. Familial skin cancer syndromes increased risk of nonmelanotic skin cancers and extracutaneous tumors. *J Am Acad Dermatol*. 2016;74(3):437–451. doi:10.1016/j.jaad.2015.08.073.

7. NCCN. National Comprehensive Cancer Network (NCCN). https://www.nccn.org/professionals/physician_gls/pdf/nmsc.pdf. Accessed August 15, 2020.

8. Gunaratne DA, Veness MJ. Efficacy of hypofractionated radiotherapy in patients with non-melanoma skin cancer: results of a systematic review. *J Med Imag Radiat Oncol*. 2018;62(3):401–411. doi:10.1111/1754–9485.12718.

9. Garbutcheon-Singh KB, Veness MJ. The role of radiotherapy in the management of non-melanoma skin cancer. *Australas J Dermatol*. 2019;60(4):265–272. doi:10.1111/ajd.13025.

10. FDA. *FDA Approves First Treatment for Advanced Form Of The Second Most Common Skin Cancer*. 2018. FDA. https://www.fda.gov/news-events/press-announcements/fda-approves-first-treatment-advanced-form-second-most-common-skin-cancer. Accessed September 6, 2020.

Case 2.1

Authors: Nicole Patzelt, MD, Sara Al Janahi MD, MSc, Iman Fatima Khan, MS, MPH, and Michael R. Cassidy, MD.

Reason for Presentation: The role of sentinel lymph node biopsy (SLNB) in cSCC.

Chief Complaint: Lump on the right arm.

History of Present Illness: An HIV-positive patient presented with a 4-month history of a painful, rapidly growing bleeding mass on the right arm. The patient denied any preceding trauma to the area. A recent 1-month course of flucloxacillin 500 mg daily in the home country outside of the United States had no therapeutic effect on the mass.

Review of Systems: No pertinent positives.

Medical/Surgical History: HIV positive.

Medications: Lamivudine/zidovudine 150–300 mg daily; nevirapine 200 mg daily.

Family History: No family history of skin cancer.

Physical Examination: Skin type V; Right arm: 3.0 × 3.0 cm friable, pink-red nodule, tender to palpation, and containing a 1.5 × 1.5 cm area of superficial ulceration (see Figure 2.1.1); palpable, mobile, right axillary lymphadenopathy.

Pathology: Punch biopsy of the right arm nodule (see Figure 2.1.2): Dermal islands of atypical squamous epithelium with central keratinization and necrosis (H&E, 200×); consistent with SCC, well-differentiated.

Investigations

- **Right axillary ultrasound:** Single lymph node enlarged by size criteria 3.1 × 1.0 × 1.1 with a curved central hilum.

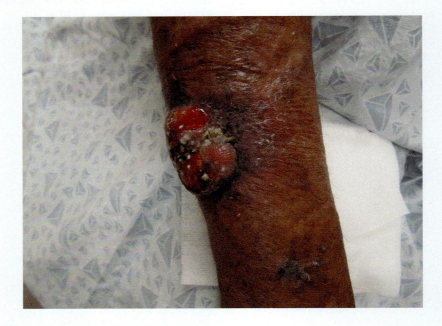

FIGURE 2.1.1   Ulcerated, friable nodule on the right arm.

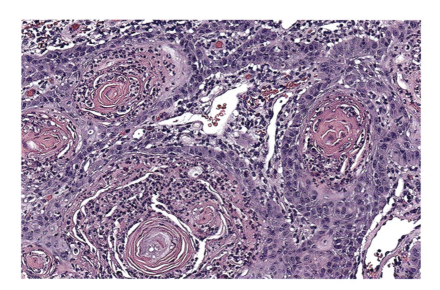

FIGURE 2.1.2 Punch biopsy from the right arm nodule: H&E, 200×.

- **CT chest, abdomen, and pelvis with contrast:** Multiple subcentimeter right axillary and subpectoralis lymph nodes that could represent metastatic disease.
- **US-guided FNA of the right axillary nodes:** No evidence of metastasis.

Final Diagnosis

- cSCC, well-differentiated, stage II (pT2cN1M0).

Management and Disease Course

- After biopsy confirmation of the patient's well-differentiated SCC, the patient was scheduled for a wide local excision (WLE) with 1 cm margins and an SLNB, given the concern regarding the lymph nodes on imaging. Although no nodal metastases were noted on the SLNB, the SCC was found to be close to the deep margin (1.5 mm from deep margin), with extension to the fascia.
- Due to the high-risk features of this patient's SCC, the decision was made to pursue adjuvant radiation, which they completed and tolerated well. The high-risk features included large tumor size >2 cm and extension to the fascial plane with proximity to the deep surgical margin (1.5 mm).

Discussion

- The vast majority of cSCCs can be cured with surgery alone, denoting an overall excellent prognosis for this cancer type. A small subset (4%–6%), however, are associated with metastasis, resulting in inferior outcomes and a mortality rate of ~2%. It is notable that cSCC accounts for ~20% of all skin cancers in the United States and is increasing in incidence.
- Identifying the subset of patients with a high risk of tumor recurrence or progression is critical as it defines patients who may benefit from nodal evaluation or adjuvant treatment. The delineation of this subset has been hampered, largely due to staging systems historically being unable to accurately stratify cSCC for this high-risk group. Part of this problem is attributed to the lack of substantial, reliable data, as cSCC are excluded from most countries' national cancer registries.

- The prior AJCC (Seventh Edition) for cSCC separated tumors based on size and/or the number of high-risk features: T1 (≤2 cm diameter with <2 high-risk features) and T2 (>2 cm diameter with or without one additional high-risk feature, or any tumor with ≥2 high-risk features). High-risk features included depth/invasion (>2 mm thickness, Clark level IV, or perineural invasion), anatomical location (primary site on the ear or the non-hair-bearing lip), and differentiation (poorly differentiated or undifferentiated). However, patients in the T2 population were found to have highly variable outcomes, and only 11.9% of T2 patients demonstrated a positive SLNB. Patients who were T3 (with bony invasion) and T4 (invasion of axial skeleton or perineural invasion of skull base) had a high rate of positive SLNB but were extremely rare in presentation. This made it difficult to effectively identify the subset of high-risk patients who might specifically benefit from a more aggressive treatment approach.[1]

- To circumvent some of the drawbacks of the AJCC (Seventh Edition), Jambusaria-Pahlajani et al. proposed an alternate staging system for cSCC in a large, single-institute study at the Brigham and Women's Hospital (BWH). They suggested removing the T4 designation and recognizing the heterogeneity of the T2 population. The authors further subdivided the T2 population into T2a (any tumor size with one risk factor) and T2b (any tumor size with 2–3 risk factors).[2] Risk factors included tumor diameter of ≥2 cm, poorly differentiated histological characteristics, perineural invasion, and tumor invasion beyond the subcutaneous fat excluding bone invasion. T3 involved patients with bone invasion. The BWH system had the advantage of identifying small tumors (<2 cm in size) that are capable of metastasizing due to other independent poor prognostic factors. The risk of nodal metastasis was found to be 0.1% in T1 disease, 3% in T2a disease, 21% in T2b disease, and 67% in T3 disease. One major drawback of the BWH staging system is that the classification of the T stage is based on two single-institution cohorts and needs validation in a more general setting.[2]

- SLNB is used to gather prognostic information in patients with certain malignancies, most commonly melanoma and breast cancer. SLNB is specifically used in patients with no palpable lymph nodes who are deemed at high risk of metastases due to tumor-related factors. Although SLNB can effectively detect micrometastases in cSCC, its role in improving survival in these patients is yet to be determined as there are no randomized controlled studies assessing this. The population group in cSCC who will benefit the most from undergoing an SLNB is also not well-characterized. In a systematic review analysis, the BWH staging system was found to be a better predictor of SLNB positivity than the AJCC (Seventh Edition). Additionally, the BWH system demonstrated sentinel node positivity in ~35% of patients meeting T2b and T3 criteria.[3] Nodal staging provides important prognostic information in cSCC. Studies show that 5-year disease-specific survival is markedly diminished in those with distant disease (11%) versus those with nodal disease (83%). Therefore, patients with metastases limited to nodal disease may have a critical window of opportunity where early intervention can improve clinical outcome. Additionally, a high 5-year survival rate of >90% can be achieved when conventional treatments are applied to patients who have microscopic metastases, underscoring the importance of identifying this population.[4]

- In 2018, the AJCC came up with an eighth edition for cSCC with reclassification of the tumors presenting in the head and neck region only. This demonstrated improved monotonicity (worsening outcomes with increasing categories) and homogeneity (similar outcomes within each category) than the AJCC (Seventh Edition).[5] In the eighth edition, tumor diameter is the main delineating factor between stages T1–T3. Thus, T1-diameter <2 cm; T2-diameter 2–3.9 cm; T3-diameter ≥4 cm, or minor bone erosion, or perineural invasion, or deep invasion; T4-involves major bone invasion. Stage T2 or higher are likely to have worse outcomes and may benefit from further work up of the nodal basin with imaging and/or SLNB. The advantage of the AJCC (Eighth Edition) is that it is based on studies performed after 2010, which outline the most relevant risk factors. The expansion of the T3 category enables greater representation of patients, including those with likely poor outcomes. However, being relatively new, the AJCC (Eighth Edition) needs validation of its prognostic accuracy.

- In a cohort study of 459 patients with 680 head and neck cSCCs from a single tertiary institution, staging was performed using both the AJCC (Eighth Edition) and the BWH system.[6] The goal of the study was to compare poor outcomes and hence the accuracy and validity of the two staging systems. The results suggested that the BWH system may have a higher specificity and positive predictive value for identifying patients at risk of nodal metastases or disease-specific death ($P = 0.1$ and $P = 0.05$, respectively).[6] The study also showed that due to better risk stratification, the BWH system was able to identify a smaller, more specific population with worse outcomes when compared to the AJCC (Eighth Edition) (9% vs. 23% of patients, respectively). As a result, the BWH system may allow for better delineation of the group that would benefit most from SLNB, thereby reducing procedural morbidity and healthcare costs by decreasing the number of unnecessary SLNBs.[6]

- Based on the above data, it may be applicable to consider nodal staging in patients who are T2b or higher in the BWH staging system. Studies are presently limited regarding radiologic nodal staging specific to cSCC, which leads to variability in clinical practice. One study found that imaging altered management in 33% of patients. These patients received adjuvant radiation more often and had a lower risk of subsequent nodal metastasis than patients who were not imaged. As a result, imaging of high-risk patients should be considered, as it may improve clinical outcomes.[7,8]

- Based on a retrospective review of the literature from head and neck cSCC, pre-operative nodal staging with ultrasonography (US) may be more useful than CT or MRI.[8] US was found to have higher sensitivity, specificity, and diagnostic odds ratio when compared to the other imaging modalities.[8] Another added advantage of US is that an FNA or core biopsy can be performed immediately if an abnormal node is detected. One disadvantage however is its high operator dependency, and a limitation common to all forms of radiologic imaging is a significant rate of false negatives. This is thought to be due to an inability to detect micrometastases.[8] There is currently no data to show that the detection of early metastasis using SLNB has a superior risk-benefit ratio over radiologic imaging to make its use in high-risk cSCC more widespread. As a result, the High-Risk Squamous Cell Carcinoma Workgroup suggests performing nodal staging via imaging in high-risk patients (in the absence of clinically palpable lymph nodes), and if negative, an SLNB procedure may be justified.[8]

Teaching Pearls

- Although the majority of cSCCs have excellent treatment outcomes and prognosis, ~5% of these lesions are at a significant risk of poor outcomes, including death. Both the AJCC (Eighth Edition) and BWH staging systems may help to identify this high-risk group, thereby delineating the population who could benefit the most from undergoing nodal staging. Further validation of the accuracy of the two staging systems is still needed.

- SLNB can detect micrometastases and provide prognostic information for high-risk patients with cSCC. However, prospective studies are needed to substantiate whether detection of early nodal metastasis will significantly impact disease-free, disease-specific, and overall survival in these patients.

References

1. American Joint Committee on Cancer. Cutaneous squamous cell carcinoma and other cutaneous carcinomas. In Edge SB, Byrd DR, Compton CC, Fritz AG, Greene FL, Trotti A, eds. *AJCC Cancer Staging Manual*. 7th ed. New York, NY: Springer. 2010, pp. 301–309.
2. Jambusaria-Pahlajani A, Kanetsky PA, Karia PS, et al. Evaluation of AJCC tumor staging for cutaneous squamous cell carcinoma and a proposed alternative tumor staging system. *JAMA Dermatol*. 2013;149(4):402–410.

3. Schmitt A, Brewer J, Bordeaux J, et al. Staging for cutaneous squamous cell carcinoma as a predictor of sentinel lymph node biopsy results: meta-analysis of American joint committee on cancer criteria and a proposed alternative system. *JAMA Dermatol.* 2014;150(1):19–24.

4. Ebrahimi A, Clark JR, Lorincz BB, et al. Metastatic head and neck cutaneous squamous cell carcinoma: defining a low-risk patient. *Head Neck.* 2012;34(3):365–70. doi: 10.1002/hed.21743. PMID: 21472887.

5. Amin MB, Edge S, Greene F, et al., eds. *AJCC Cancer Staging Manual.* 8th ed. New York, NY: Springer. 2017.

6. Ruiz ES, Karia PS, Besaw R, et al. Staging for cutaneous squamous cell carcinoma as a predictor of sentinel lymph node biopsy results meta-analysis of American joint committee on cancer criteria and a proposed alternative system. *JAMA Dermatol.* 2019;155(7):819–825.

7. Que S, Zwald F, Schmults C. Cutaneous squamous cell carcinoma: incidence, risk factors, diagnosis, and staging. *J Am Acad Dermatol.* 2018;78(2):237–247.

8. Fox M, Brown M, Golda N, et al. Nodal staging of high-risk cutaneous squamous cell carcinoma. *J Am Acad Dermatol.* 2019;81(2):548–557.

Case 2.2

Authors: Sarah Ann Kam, MD, Hanna E. Mumber, BS, Malathi Chittireddy, MD, MSc, and Minh T. Truong, MD.

Reason for Presentation: cSCC treated with curative RT.

Chief Complaint: Growth on the left leg.

History of Present Illness: A nonagenarian with advanced Alzheimer's dementia presented from a nursing home with a painful, enlarging lesion on the left leg. The patient denied bleeding or drainage from this lesion. The exact duration of the lesion was unclear. There was no prior history of skin cancer.

Review of Systems: No pertinent positives.

Medical/Surgical History: End-stage renal disease, chronic heart failure, Alzheimer's disease, transient ischemic attack.

Medications: None.

Family History: No family history of cancer.

Social History: Wheelchair-bound, nursing home resident, dependent for all activities of daily living.

Physical Exam: Fitzpatrick skin type II; left popliteal fossa: 4.0 × 2.5 cm pink, well-defined, exophytic, ulcerated nodule with hemorrhagic crust (see Figure 2.2.1); bilateral lower legs: Significant pedal edema to knee level.

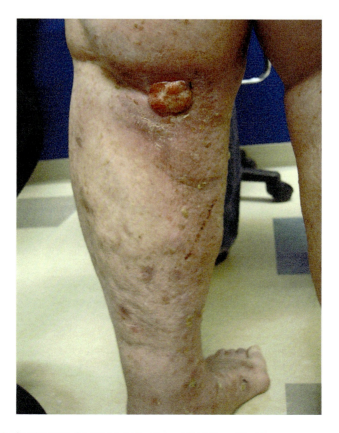

FIGURE 2.2.1   Exophytic, ulcerated, focally crusted nodule on the left popliteal fossa.

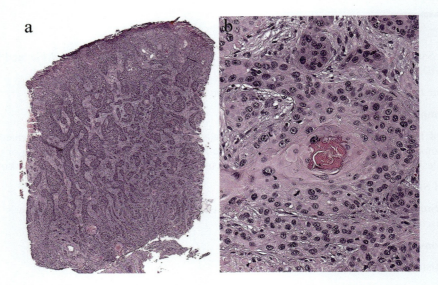

FIGURE 2.2.2   Punch biopsy from the left popliteal nodule: (a) H&E, low power and (b) H&E, high power.

Pathology: Punch biopsy of the left popliteal fossa ulcerated nodule (see Figure 2.2.2): (a) Lobules and strands of squamous epithelium infiltrating the reticular dermis (H&E, 40×), and (b) Tumor lobules composed of atypical squamous epithelium with foci of keratinization (H&E, 200×).

Final Diagnosis: Squamous cell carcinoma, moderately to well-differentiated, stage II (T2NxMx).

Management: Given the multiple comorbidities, poor general health status, and the likelihood of increased surgical complications due to venous insufficiency, the patient was deemed a non-surgical candidate. The multidisciplinary tumor board team recommended definitive radiotherapy with the goal of therapy being curative while maintaining quality of life as best as possible.

As per the NCCN guidelines, the patient received radiation treatment with a cumulative dose of 51 Gy in 17 fractions over 3 weeks, with excellent response. The patient tolerated the therapy well and completed it without any unplanned breaks. By the time the patient received 33 Gy, the ulcerated SCC looked flatter and was no longer painful. By the end of treatment, the tumor had completely resolved without any ulceration. During the course of radiation, the patient developed mild radiation dermatitis at the treatment portal. This responded to appropriate topical treatment with petrolatum and oil emulsion dressings. The patient had complete response to radiation treatment, and regular follow-up for 2 years showed no evidence of local or regional recurrence.

Discussion

- A locally advanced, large (stage T2), well-differentiated squamous cell carcinoma of the lower extremity qualifies for Mohs surgery under the "Mohs Appropriate Use Criteria".[1] In cases where surgery is likely to have significant complications and negatively impact the quality of life of a patient, definitive radiotherapy can be offered as an excellent alternative.
- Mohs surgery offers a high cure rate of up to 95% in the treatment of non-melanoma skin cancers (NMSC), as it enables complete evaluation of the surgical margin.[2] The 5-year recurrence rate of SCC treated with Mohs ranges from 0% to 4%.[3] In comparison, a retrospective analysis of NMSCs treated with superficial radiotherapy revealed a 5-year recurrence rate of approximately 6% for cSCC.[4] Thus, definitive radiotherapy provides a good alternative to surgery, and RT may be curative for both cSCC and BCC.

- External beam radiotherapy (EBRT) using superficial orthovoltage or electron beam radiotherapy to the appropriate treatment depth is the recommended treatment for NMSCs based on the history of use and available data.[5] The type of EBRT depends on the tumor size and the availability of equipment. For flat small lesions of less than 5 mm depth, superficial X-rays may be adequate, but for deeper lesions, orthovoltage or electron beam therapy is used. Orthovoltage therapy has the advantage of being able to collimate the beam on the skin with a sharp penumbra, so the maximum dose is at the skin surface. There is skin sparing with electron beam therapy, with lower electron energies having higher skin sparing. Hence, a tissue equivalent bolus would be required to ensure adequate dose to the tumor when using electron beam therapy.

- For deeper tumors (3–5 cm), megavoltage therapy using photons is preferred. In cases where there is perineural invasion with a named nerve, photons with intensity modulated radiotherapy may be the best method to adequately cover the gross tumor and any elective areas of potential spread.[5]

- Relative contraindications to the use of radiation include a previously radiated tumor, patients with connective tissue diseases such as scleroderma, or lupus, and peripheral vascular disease.[4]

- Common side effects of radiotherapy include radiation dermatitis, post-inflammatory hyper/hypopigmentation, soft tissue fibrosis, microvascular changes in the subcutaneous tissue, and underlying arterial vessel narrowing. Radiation dermatitis can be treated with emollients and topical steroids, although some inflammatory response to radiotherapy is thought to be beneficial. Delaying or pausing treatment is generally avoided due to the possibility of accelerated repopulation of tumor cells. However, it may be warranted in the event of significant moist desquamation or ulceration.[5]

Teaching Pearls

- Although Mohs surgery is favored as the first-line treatment for high-risk SCC, RT can produce comparable outcomes (~6% recurrent rate for radiation vs. ~0%–4% for Mohs).
- RT is an effective and safe alternative to surgery for the treatment of SCCs in non-surgical candidates or for those who wish to avoid surgery. This modality may be considered in cosmetically sensitive areas close to the eyes or nose and has an excellent outcome.

References

1. Ad Hoc Task Force, Connolly SM, Baker DR, et al. AAD/ACMS/ASDSA/ASMS 2012 appropriate use criteria for Mohs micrographic surgery: a report of the American Academy of Dermatology, American College of Mohs Surgery, American Society for Dermatologic Surgery Association, and the American Society for Mohs Surgery. *J Am Acad Dermatol*. 2012;67(4):531–550. doi:10.1016/j.jaad.2012.06.009.
2. Cohen DK, Goldberg DJ. Mohs micrographic surgery: past, present, and future. *Dermatol Surg*. 2019;45(3):329–339. doi:10.1097/DSS.0000000000001701.
3. Chren M-M, Linos E, Torres JS, et al. Tumor recurrence 5 years after treatment of cutaneous basal cell carcinoma and squamous cell carcinoma. *J Invest Dermatol*. 2013;133(5):1188–1196. doi:10.1038/jid.2012.403.
4. Nestor MS, Berman B, Goldberg D, et al. Consensus guidelines on the use of superficial radiation therapy for treating nonmelanoma skin cancers and keloids. *J Clin Aesthetic Dermatol*. 2019;12(2):12–18.
5. Cognetta AB, Howard BM, Heaton HP, et al. Superficial x-ray in the treatment of basal and squamous cell carcinomas: a viable option in select patients. *J Am Acad Dermatol*. 2012;67(6):1235–1241. doi:10.1016/j.jaad.2012.06.001.

Case 2.3

Authors: Marguerite Sullivan, MD, Malathi Chittireddy, MD, MSc, Hannah E. Mumber, BS, and Waleed Ezzat, MD, FACS.

Reason for Presentation: Advanced cSCC in a renal transplant patient.

Chief Complaint: Lesion on the right temple.

History of Present Illness: A middle-aged patient with a history of scleroderma and kidney transplant presented to the dermatologist for evaluation of a rapidly growing bump on the right temple. The lesion was intermittently painful and would bleed spontaneously. There was no personal history of skin cancer, and the patient reported three to five blistering sunburns in childhood.

Review of Systems: No pertinent positives.

Medical/Surgical History: Systemic sclerosis, end-stage renal disease s/p cadaveric kidney transplant 3 years prior to above presentation.

Relevant Medications: Tacrolimus, azathioprine, prednisone.

Family History: No family history of skin cancer.

Physical Examination: Right anterior temple: 1.2 × 1.2 cm erythematous nodule with central hemorrhagic crust (see Figure 2.3.1); Cheeks and nasal dorsum: Multiple matted telangiectasias; no palpable auricular or cervical adenopathy.

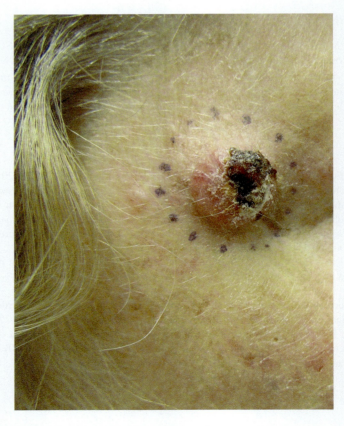

FIGURE 2.3.1   Centrally crusted nodule on the right anterior temple.

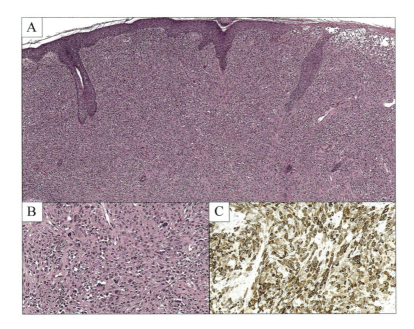

FIGURE 2.3.2 Incisional biopsy from the right anterior temple: (A) H&E, low power; (B) H&E, high power; and (C) high-molecular-weight cytokeratin immunostain.

Pathology: Incisional biopsy, right anterior temple nodule (see Figure 2.3.2); (A) A diffuse dermal proliferation of atypical cells (H&E, 40×); (B) Higher power revealing pleomorphism with plasmacytoid (arrow) and focally binucleate cells (arrowhead) (H&E, 200×); and (C) Lesional cells positive for high-molecular-weight cytokeratin (34betaE12, 200×).

Final Diagnosis: Poorly differentiated cSCC.

Management and Disease Course: Based on the high-risk features (immunosuppression, rapidly growing tumor, poorly differentiated cSCC), the patient was referred for Mohs micrographic surgery. Even after six stages of Mohs, the margins remained positive for cSCC. The patient was referred to head and neck surgical oncology, and within a period of 2 weeks underwent a WLE with right eye lid excision, right parotidectomy, and right level 1–3 neck dissection. Unfortunately, even this re-excision was positive for cancer at the margins, and one of the lymph nodes sampled came back positive for metastatic cSCC with extranodal extension. Additionally, the patient was noted to have developed new skin-colored satellite nodules a few centimeters away from the location of the primary tumor (see Figure 2.3.3). One of these nodules was sampled at the time of WLE and was confirmed to be cutaneous in-transit metastasis of cSCC. Further surgery was impractical due to the extent of locoregional disease. Following a limited reconstruction with a split-thickness skin graft, the patient was referred for adjuvant radiation which was completed successfully.

  Tacrolimus was switched to everolimus in an effort to enhance the patient's immune response to his cSCC. Immune checkpoint therapy was also considered given the highly aggressive nature of the patient's tumor. The patient was counseled extensively, and it was made apparent that this therapy would put the patient at a high risk of kidney rejection and associated morbidity. Conversely, the patient clearly had a highly aggressive metastatic cSCC with a poor prognosis. At the time of presentation, there was no FDA-approved immunotherapy for advanced cSCC. However, data from several case reports suggested this could be therapeutically successfully in select cases. After being presented with this difficult choice, the patient opted to forego immune checkpoint therapy. Soon thereafter, the patient developed shortness of breath and hospital admission identified extensive lung metastases. This was followed by rapid clinical deterioration, and the patient succumbed to the illness.

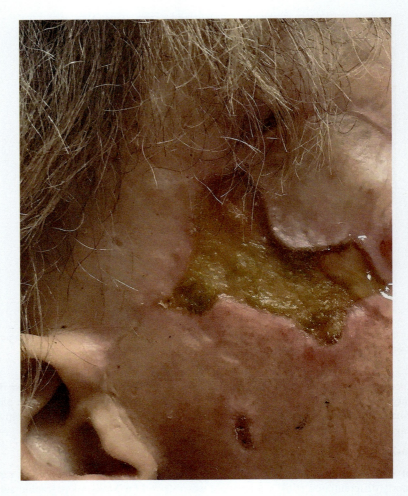

FIGURE 2.3.3 Large healing surgical scar with fibrinous crust; surrounding the scar, multiple irregular pink skin-colored papulonodules can be seen on the right temple and cheek.

Discussion

- Organ transplant recipients (OTRs) are at an increased risk of malignancy, most commonly skin cancer. cSCC and BCC make up the greatest proportion of these malignancies, but Kaposi's sarcoma, melanoma, and Merkel cell carcinoma are also increased in these patients. cSCCs in OTRs are often aggressive with poor prognostic features, higher recurrence rates, and increased risk of metastases and death.[1] Decreased immune-mediated tumor surveillance due to life-long immunosuppression plays a large role in the increased risk of malignancy. Age, cumulative sun exposure, as well as dose, duration, and type of immunosuppressive medication also contribute. Azathioprine, calcineurin inhibitors, and prednisolone have been associated with an increased risk of cSCC. Mycophenolate mofetil has been shown to have a lower risk of photocarcinogenesis than azathioprine.[2]

- mTOR inhibitors sirolimus and everolimus have been associated with a lower risk of skin malignancies in solid OTRs when compared to calcineurin inhibitors. The lower risk has been attributed to the fact that mTOR inhibitors have both immunosuppressive and anti-neoplastic activity. Consistent with this observation, when patients with renal transplants develop Kaposi's sarcoma, a switch from calcineurin inhibitor-based immune suppression to the mTOR inhibitor sirolimus is frequently associated with tumor regression.[3] While the mechanism is not fully understood, partial reconstitution of the host T-cells' ability to combat the malignancy is thought to contribute to improved outcomes, as well as the direct anti-neoplastic effect of reducing mTOR signaling in tumors.[4,5] However, mTOR inhibitors are certainly not without potential side effects, most notably delayed wound healing. Therefore, such a transition in immunosuppression should only be made in conjunction with the renal transplant physicians who oversee the patient's immunosuppressive medications.[4,6]

- The data on the use of immune checkpoint therapy in renal transplant recipients are limited as most of these patients were excluded from the initial clinical trials due to the theoretical risk of graft rejection, in which T-cells play a significant role.[7,8] In the limited number of cases reported to date of renal transplant patients treated with checkpoint therapy, kidney rejection occurred in 40%–45%. Graft rejection was the highest in nivolumab (52%), followed by pembrolizumab (26.7%) and ipilimumab (25%), though an association between the specific type of medication and graft rejection was not found to be statistically significant. The overall response rate of cSCC to immune checkpoint inhibition has been promising, with pembrolizumab demonstrating the highest response rate (40%), followed by nivolumab (30%) and ipilimumab (25%). In the majority of patients, death was due to progression of malignancy rather than graft failure.[7,8]

Teaching Pearls

- OTRs are at an increased risk of cutaneous malignancy, most commonly cSCC. Additionally, cSCCs are more likely to behave aggressively with an increased risk of recurrence and metastases.
- In patients with cSCCs that develop in the setting of a prior solid organ transplant, calcineurin inhibitor-based immunosuppression is usually switched to an mTOR inhibitor, such as sirolimus, in conjunction with the renal transplant team.
- While anti-PD-1-based immune checkpoint inhibition may be quite clinically active in transplant-associated cSCC, it carries a substantial risk of graft rejection, and the decision to proceed with such therapy will vary according to the patient's preferences.

References

1. Mittal A, Colegio OR. Skin cancers in organ transplant recipients. *Am J Transpl.* 2017;17:2509.
2. Howard M, Su D, Chong J. Skin cancer following solid organ transplantation: a review of risk factors and models of care. *Am J Clin Dermatol.* 2018;19(4):585–597.
3. Knoll GA, Kokolo MB, Mallick R, et al. Effect of sirolimus on malignancy and survival after kidney transplantation: systematic review and meta-analysis of individual patient data. *BMJ.* 2014;349:6679.
4. Dharnidharka VR, Schnitzler MA, Chen J, et al. Differential risks for adverse outcomes 3 years after kidney transplantation based on initial immunosuppression regimen: a national study. *Transpl Int.* 2016;29:1226.
5. Dharnidharka VR, Schnitzler MA, Chen J, et al. Differential risks for adverse outcomes 3 years after kidney transplantation based on initial immunosuppression regimen: a national study. *Transpl Int.* 2016;29:1226.
6. De Bruyn P, Van Gestel D, Ost P, et al. Immune checkpoint blockade for organ transplant patients with advanced cancer: how far can we go? *Curr Opin Oncol.* 2019;31(2):54–64. doi:10.1097/CCO.0000000000000505.
7. Fisher J, Zeitouni N, Fan W, et al. Immune checkpoint inhibitor therapy in solid organ transplant recipients: a patient-centered systematic review. *J Am Acad Dermatol.* 2020;82(6):1490–1500.

Case 2.4

Authors: Bilal Fawaz, MD, Marguerite Sullivan, MD, Sara Al Janahi MD, MSc, Iman Fatima Khan, MS, MPH, and Adam Lerner, MD.

Reason for Presentation: The use of PD-1 inhibitors to treat advanced cSCC.

Chief Complaint: Growth on the right forehead.

History of Present Illness: An older patient with a history of chronic sun damage presented with a painless, enlarging mass on the right forehead. The mass appeared 1 year ago as a small "sore". It progressively enlarged and began to drain a yellow, malodorous discharge, which prompted the patient to see the dermatologist.

Review of Systems: No pertinent positives.

Medical/Surgical History: None.

Medications: None.

Social History: Worked outdoors throughout life.

Family History: No family history of cancer.

Physical Examination: Fitzpatrick skin type I; Right temple: A 7.0 × 7.5 × 1.0 cm thick, indurated, pink tumor with central necrosis, full-thickness ulceration, and foul-smelling discharge (see Figure 2.4.1). A similar appearing lesion was also noted on the dorsum of the right hand.

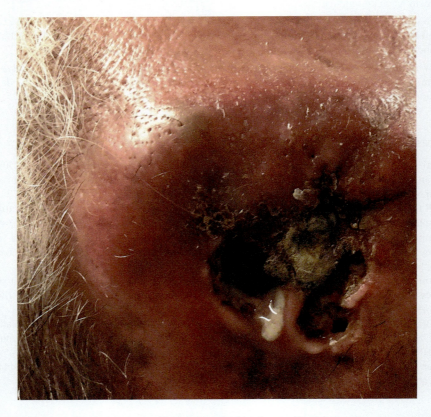

FIGURE 2.4.1 Large erythematous tumor with central cavitating ulcer on the right temple, encroaching on the right upper eyelid.

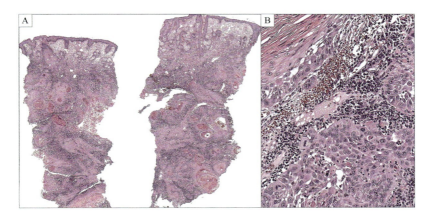

FIGURE 2.4.2 Punch biopsy of the right temple tumor: (A) H&E, low power and (B) H&E, high power.

Pathology: Punch biopsy of the right temple nodule (see Figure 2.4.2): (A) Eosinophilic epithelial tumor filling the dermis (H&E, 10×), and (B) Higher power revealing aggregates of atypical acantholytic squamous epithelium with a surrounding lymphoplasmacytic infiltrate and extensive areas of keratinization (H&E, 200×).

Investigations: Imaging was carried out to both stage the cancer, and given the pathology report, to rule out the possibility of the skin lesions being secondary cutaneous metastases from a primary visceral SCC.

- **MRI of brain with and without contrast:** Involvement by the soft tissue mass of the right temporalis muscle, right pterygoid muscle, lacrimal gland, superior eyelid, lateral canthus, frontotemporal skull, possible trigeminal nerve, and several enlarged right cervical lymph nodes.
- **CT of neck, abdomen, pelvis with contrast:** No evidence of a primary visceral malignancy.

Final Diagnosis: Moderately to well-differentiated primary cSCC on the right temple and the dorsum of the right hand.

Management: The patient was presented at the cutaneous oncology tumor board. Surgical excision was deemed to be problematic and unlikely to result in a cure given the extensive local and regional spread on imaging. The morbidity from surgery was likely to exceed its benefits. Radiation with adjuvant cetuximab was felt to be palliative, and given the close proximity of the cSCC to the right eye, was anticipated to cause loss of functioning vision. At the time of presentation of this patient, there was no FDA-approved systemic therapy for advanced cSCC. However, based on growing literature supporting the use of PD-1 inhibitors in unresectable cSCC, pembrolizumab off-label use was advised by the tumor board panel at a dose of 2 mg/kg every 21 days.

   After the first infusion, the patient was noted to develop painless right axillary lymphadenopathy. Given the rapid presentation and known side effects of the medication, immune-related pseudo-progression was suspected as the cause. The team continued treatment with close monitoring and without further investigation. As expected, the lymph nodes fully resolved within 2 months. Marked clinical improvement of the two cSCCs was noted by the third infusion with complete clinical and radiological resolution of both lesions by the ninth infusion (see Figure 2.4.3). Pembrolizumab was discontinued after a total of 12 months of therapy. Close clinical monitoring with repeat interval imaging showed no evidence of disease recurrence 2 years following completion of treatment. The patient tolerated the treatment well, with mild fatigue only.

Discussion

- cSCC is the second most common skin cancer, typically cured with surgical excision in more than 95% of cases. In contrast, rarer cases of locally advanced and metastatic cSCC pose a

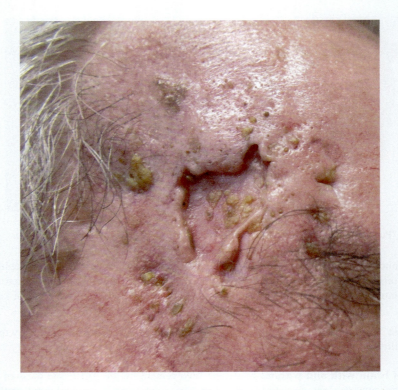

FIGURE 2.4.3 Complete clinical regression of the tumor with scarring and fibrosis on the right temple.

therapeutic challenge with limited effective treatment options until recently. Prior treatment approaches included platinum-based chemotherapy and off-label use of the EGFR inhibitor, cetuximab, with radiotherapy. However, responses to these therapies are typically not durable, with a 5-year survival rate of less than 40% for advanced cSCC. Additionally, cSCC is mostly a disease of older individuals with multiple comorbidities who frequently may have difficulty tolerating these systemic agents.[1]

- Cumulative clinical and preclinical data have suggested that the immune system plays an important role in the evolution of cSCC. Immunosuppressed transplant patients have a 65–250-fold higher risk of developing cSCC compared to the general population. This patient group is also at a greater risk of aggressive cSCCs that are more likely to recur and metastasize (see Case 2.3). On a related note, precursors of cSCC have been shown to respond well to immune modulators, such as imiquimod, a Toll-like receptor 7 agonist.[1]

- Molecular studies have shown that PD-L1 expression is significantly increased in the tumor microenvironment of cSCC when compared to precursor lesions of cSCC, which, in turn, show greater PD-L1 expression than normal skin. Additionally, cSCC are packed with tumor-infiltrating lymphocytes (TILs), and immunohistochemistry staining has localized PD-L1 staining to these TILs, even more than the tumor cells themselves. Researchers have also demonstrated a correlation between the level of PD-L1 expression in cSCC and the biological behavior of the cancer. PD-L1 expression is greater in high-risk cSCC and in cSCC metastases compared to low-risk cSCC. The level of expression of membranous PD-L1 expression in tumor cells and/or in TILs within the tumor microenvironment can help to predict the response to PD-1 antibody treatment in several cancers, with greater PD-L1 expression correlating with better treatment response.[2,4]

- Tumor mutation burden (TMB) of cancers can be measured by targeted comprehensive genomic profiling (CGP) assays and exome sequencing. When comparing TMB in a diverse cohort of cancers, skin cancers were found to have some of the highest TMB, with cSCC having the highest. This association is known to be due to UV irradiation-induced transition mutations at dipyrimidine sequences containing cytosine. A high TMB is recently emerging as an important biomarker to predict the response of a cancer to immune checkpoint therapy with PD-1 and PD-L1 inhibitors. Having both high TMB and high PD-L1 expression in cSCC suggested a potential role for PD-1 inhibitors in the treatment of advanced cSCC. These observations formed the basis for the off-label use of pembrolizumab for advanced cSCC and led to a number of published case reports, as well as the choice of this drug in our patient.[5,6]

- Subsequent to the presentation of our case, another anti-PD-1 antibody, cemiplimab, was approved by the FDA in 2018 for the treatment of unresectable advanced and metastatic cutaneous SCC. This medication was shown to induce durable responses in phase I and II clinical trials with a 47% response rate (95% CI, 34–61) and a durable response rate of 61% (95% CI, 47–74). Among the patients who responded, 57% had a response lasting greater than 6 months and approximately 80% had ongoing responses after the trial ended. Cemiplimab had comparable overall responses in both locally advanced cSCC and those with metastatic disease; a response was observed in 6 of 14 patients with regional metastasis (43%; 95% CI, 18–71) and in 22 of 45 patients with distant metastases (49%; 95% CI, 34–64). Side effects of cemiplimab were similar to other immune checkpoint inhibitors, including diarrhea, fatigue, nausea, and rash. Importantly, the drug was well-tolerated in patients of advanced age.[7]

- Our case demonstrated pseudo-progression early on in treatment. This is an uncommon phenomenon where the tumor enlarges and appears to progress. However, the increase in size is due to the checkpoint inhibitor causing a sudden influx of inflammatory cells into the tumor, resulting in a temporary increase in tumor size prior to subsequent shrinkage. Such pseudo-progression was seen in 3 of 16 patients in the phase I trial of cemiplimab, and it is important to recognize to avoid discontinuing therapy prematurely.

Teaching Pearls

- This case provides an example of an advanced cSCC where both surgery and radiation were thought to likely be associated with unacceptable morbidity and little chance of cure. The approved anti-PD-1 agents cemiplimab and off-label pembrolizumab provide an effective, alternative first-line therapy for advanced cSCC with significant potential for a durable response.
- The drugs are generally well-tolerated, even in populations of advanced age.
- Pseudo-progression is an uncommon but well-recognized phenomenon that clinicians should be aware of when using checkpoint inhibitors.

References

1. Que, SKT, Zwald FO, Schmults CD, Cutaneous squamous cell carcinoma: management of advanced and high-stage tumors. *J Am Acad Dermatol.* 2018;78(2):249–261.
2. Gambichler T, Gnielka M, Rüddel I, et al. Expression of PD-L1 in keratoacanthoma and different stages of progression in cutaneous squamous cell carcinoma. *Cancer Immunol Immunother.* 2017;66(9):1199–1204.
3. Stevenson ML, Wang CQ, Abikhair M, et al. Expression of programmed cell death ligand in cutaneous squamous cell carcinoma and treatment of locally advanced disease with pembrolizumab. *JAMA Dermatol.* 2017;153(4):299–303.
4. Chalmers ZR, Connelly CF, Fabrizio D, et al. Analysis of 100,000 human cancer genomes reveals the landscape of tumor mutational burden. *Genome Med.* 2017;9(1):34.
5. Goodman AM, Kato S, Bazhenova L, et al. Tumor mutational burden as an independent predictor of response to immunotherapy in diverse cancers. *Mol Cancer Ther.* 2017;16(11):2598–2608.
6. Migden MR, Rischin D, Schmults C, et al. PD-1 blockade with cemiplimab in advanced cutaneous squamous-cell carcinoma. *N Engl J Med.* 2018;379(4):341–351.

Case 2.5

Authors: Nicole Patzelt, MD, Bilal Fawaz, MD, and Waleed Ezzat, MD, FACS.

Reason for Presentation: Advanced cSCC in the setting of epidermodysplasia verruciformis (EDV).

Chief Complaint: Ulcer on the forehead.

History of Present Illness: A young patient presented with a 2.5-year history of an asymptomatic growth on the right forehead. The lesion grew slowly from onset and became painful with purulent drainage. As it enlarged, it started to encroach on the right eye field of vision, which prompted the patient to see a physician. Of note, the patient also had an asymptomatic but widespread rash affecting the trunk and arms for more than 15 years. The patient's siblings also had a similar rash since childhood, but they had not sought medical help for this.

Review of Systems: No pertinent positives.

Medical/Surgical History: None.

Medications: None.

Family History: No family history of skin cancer.

Physical Examination: Right lateral forehead: Solitary 7.0 × 5.0 cm ulcerated tumor with a pink base, foci of central necrosis, and overlying serous crust (see Figure 2.5.1); Right frontoparietal scalp: Three

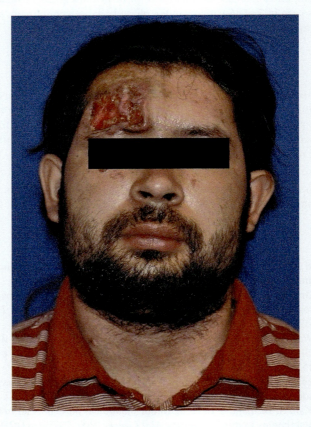

FIGURE 2.5.1 Pre-operative appearance of the ulcerated tumor on the right lateral forehead. Note the extent of the ulcerative lesion encroaching on the brow and upper lid subunits of the face. The deep end of the mass was intimately involved with the pericranium requiring excision of this layer and the adjacent outer cortical layer of the frontal bone.

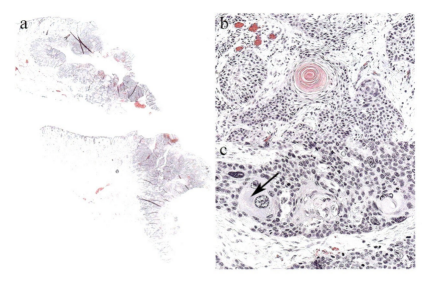

FIGURE 2.5.2 Punch biopsy of the right lateral forehead tumor: (a) H&E, 10×; (b) H&E, 100×; and (c) H&E, 200×.

discrete 0.8–1 cm well-circumscribed, shiny, erythematous, pink/purple dermal papules; Left forehead: 0.8 cm well-circumscribed shiny erythematous pink/purple telangiectatic dermal papule; Chest, abdomen, and upper back: Light pink slightly atrophic finely scaly thin papules and small patches; Dorsal hands, feet, arms, and legs with over 100 flat-topped 4–6 mm, thin verrucous pink papules, admixed with multiple light pink slightly atrophic finely scaly thin papules.

Pathology: Punch biopsy of the right lateral forehead tumor (see Figure 2.5.2). (a) A deeply infiltrative tumor arising from the epidermis (H&E, 10×). (b) Lobules of focally keratinizing squamous epithelium (H&E, 100×). (c) Higher power revealing a cell with copious blue-gray cytoplasm (arrow), consistent with EDV (H&E, 200×).

Investigations

- Rapid plasma reagin (RPR) and HIV testing was negative.
- CT head demonstrated a 6 × 5 × 1 cm ulcerated mass overlying the right frontal bone, extending over the right lateral orbital rim with attenuation higher than subcutaneous fat; no abnormal vessels noted; associated hyperostosis of the outer cortex of the frontal bone was also noted.

Final Diagnosis: Squamous cell carcinoma, moderate to well-differentiated, in the setting of EDV.

Management and Disease Course: Based on the high-risk features of this cSCC (>2 mm thickness, >2 cm diameter, reaching subcutaneous tissues, high-risk anatomic area), the patient was treated with a WLE, an SLNB, and adjuvant radiation. The defect was reconstructed using a radial forearm free tissue transplant (see Figures 2.5.3 and 2.5.4). Although no perineural invasion was noted on pathology, invasion of the right facial nerve frontal branch was presumed given the patient had an immobile right frontalis muscle with local ulceration pre-operatively. SLNB was negative and reconstruction was performed using a radial forearm auto-tissue transplant.

   The patient had a good response to this treatment but continued to develop many lesions consistent with hypertrophic AK and SCCis. For skin cancer prevention, nicotinamide 500 mg BID and low-dose acitretin 10 mg daily were started. Despite the short follow-up interval of 1 year (as the patient was lost to follow-up), the patient developed fewer SCCs in this time period in comparison to before the initiation of these medications.

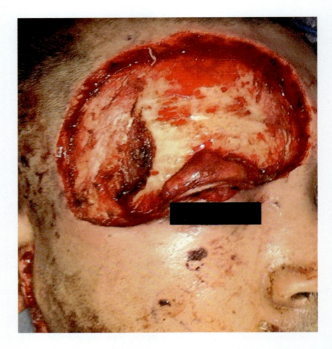

FIGURE 2.5.3   The extent of the patient's defect after WLE and before reconstruction using a radial forearm free tissue transplant.

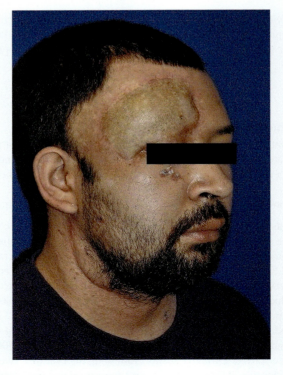

FIGURE 2.5.4   Post-operative appearance of the patient after 10 months. Note the recent excision of a new SCC is on the right cheek.

Discussion

- Patients at high risk of developing cSCC are ideal candidates for skin cancer chemoprevention. Agents such as low-dose acitretin (0.2–0.4 mg/kg/day) or nicotinamide (500 mg BID) represent a generally well-tolerated approach to skin cancer prevention.[1,2]

- EDV is a rare genodermatosis associated with widespread recalcitrant verrucae.[4] The warts are caused by certain human papillomavirus (HPV) strains, most notably HPV-5 and HPV-8.[4] It is autosomal recessive and has been associated with mutations in the *EVER1* and *EVER2* genes.[4] The mutations result in defects in cellular immunity, resulting in the patients' characteristic susceptibility to HPV infections.[4]

- Patients often present in childhood with flat-topped, skin-colored to pink papules and coalescent hypopigmented macules and patches, primarily affecting the trunk. Lesions can also develop on the head, neck, and extremities.[4] EDV patients are at a higher risk of developing NMSC, particularly SCC. This most commonly begins in the fourth decade of life and occurs in about 60% of patients.[4] HPV-5 and HPV-8 have been isolated in up to 90% of cSCCs from EDV patients.[5] As a result, minimizing other risk factors that contribute to skin cancer development is essential in this patient population.

- In addition to sun-protective measures, acitretin has been studied as a method of skin cancer chemoprevention.[6,7] Bavinck et al. demonstrated that renal transplant patients placed on a 6-month treatment regimen of acitretin 30 mg daily developed significantly fewer cSCCs than the control group (11% vs. 47%, respectively).[6] Overall, 2/19 patients in the treatment group each developed a single cSCC, whereas there was a total of 18 new cSCC diagnoses in the control group.[6]

- Kadakia et al. studied the use of acitretin for skin cancer chemoprevention in non-transplant patients.[7] Patients were placed on a 2-year treatment regimen of acitretin 25 mg 5 days a week. Although no statistically significant reduction in the rate of new cSCC was noted (odds ratio, 0.41; 95% CI, 0.15–1.13; $P = 0.13$), their data showed a trend that favored acitretin use when accounting for all NMSCs.[7]

- Acitretin was fairly well-tolerated in both of these studies. Side effects experienced included mucocutaneous side effects, mild hair loss, increases in serum cholesterol or triglycerides, and liver function abnormalities.[6,7]

- Nicotinamide has also been investigated as another option for skin cancer chemoprevention. Chen et al. evaluated 386 patients with a history of at least two NMSCs in the prior 5 years.[8] At 12 months, participants who received nicotinamide 500 mg twice daily developed significantly fewer BCC and cSCC compared to the placebo group (20% and 30%, respectively).[8] The overall rate reduction for NMSC was 23%, and no adverse effects were noted with nicotinamide use.[8] It is important to ensure the patient does not substitute nicotinamide for niacin. The latter is associated with uncomfortable facial flushing, whereas nicotinamide is not.

- Celecoxib, a cyclooxygenase 2 inhibitor, is another potential agent that may be effective in skin cancer chemoprevention.[9] A randomized controlled trial involving 240 patients evaluated its efficacy in reducing the number of actinic keratoses and NMSCs, after animal studies indicated that cyclooxygenase-2 is essential in UV-induced skin cancer.[9] After 9 months of therapy with 200 mg of celecoxib twice daily or placebo, a significantly lower rate of NMSC was noted in the treatment group compared to the control group (rate ratio of 0.41, 95% CI, 0.23–0.72; $P = 0.002$).[9] The rate of adverse events was comparable in both groups, including that of cardiovascular events, and no deaths were reported.[9]

Teaching Pearls

- Patients with EDV are at a high risk of developing SCC due to their inherited suscepti-bility to HPV infections. Regular skin checks and skin cancer prevention therapies are important in their management.
- In patients at high risk for developing SCC, chemoprevention can help decrease the number of new SCC diagnoses. Nicotinamide 500 mg twice daily and celecoxib 200 mg twice daily are relatively well-tolerated methods of skin cancer chemoprevention. Long-term acitretin (0.2–0.4 mg/kg/day) can also be considered for chemoprevention in patients at high risk of SCC but requires blood monitoring.

References

1. Harwood CA, Leedham-Green M, Leigh IM, et al. Low-dose retinoids in the prevention of cutaneous squamous cell carcinomas in organ transplant recipients: a 16-year retrospective study. *Arch Dermatol.* 2005;141(4):456–464.
2. Minocha R, Damian DL, Halliday GM. Melanoma and nonmelanoma skin cancer chemoprevention: a role for nicotinamide?. *Photodermatol Photoimmunol Photomed.* 2018;34(1):5–12.
3. Stallone G, Schena A, Infante B, et al. Sirolimus for Kaposi's sarcoma in renal-transplant recipients. *New England Journal of Medicine.* 2005;352:1317–1323.
4. Fox SH, Elston DM. Epidermodysplasia verruciformis and the risk for malignancy. *Cutis.* 2016;98(4):E10–E12.
5. Accardi R, Gheit T. Cutaneous HPV and skin cancer. *Presse Med.* 2014;43(12 Pt 2):e435–e443.
6. Bavinck JN, Tieben LM, Van der Woude FJ, et al. Prevention of skin cancer and reduction of keratotic skin lesions during acitretin therapy in renal transplant recipients: a double-blind, placebo-controlled study. *J Clin Oncol.* 1995;13(8):1933–1938.
7. Kadakia KC, Barton DL, Loprinzi CL, et al. Randomized controlled trial of acitretin versus placebo in patients at high risk for basal cell or squamous cell carcinoma of the skin (North Central Cancer Treatment Group Study 969251). *Cancer.* 2012;118(8):2128–2137.
8. Chen AC, Martin AJ, Choy B, et al. A phase 3 randomized trial of nicotinamide for skin-cancer chemo-prevention. *N Engl J Med.* 2015;373(17):1618–1626.
9. Elmets CA, Viner JL, Pentland AP, et al. Chemoprevention of nonmelanoma skin cancer with celecoxib: a randomized, double-blind, placebo-controlled trial. *J Natl Cancer Inst.* 2010;102(24):1835–1844. doi:10.1093/jnci/djq442.

3

Basal Cell Carcinoma

Ali Al-Haseni and Debjani Sahni

CONTENTS

Introduction

Cutaneous carcinomas are the most common type of malignancies, with incidence increasing steadily over time due to an aging world population.[1] Basal cell carcinoma (BCC) is a slow-growing, locally destructive cancer with a low risk of metastasis.[2] It tends to appear on chronically sun-exposed areas of the body. Untreated, it can grow to several centimeters in size, causing ulcers with local destruction. Multiple therapeutic options exist, but surgery continues to be the gold standard curative modality.[2]

BCC is the most common carcinoma in fair-skinned individuals, and is the most common malignancy in humans, with an incidence of more than 1,000 per 100,000 person-years in Australia.[2,3] The exact incidence of BCC in the United States is difficult to calculate as non-melanoma skin cancers are not reported to cancer registries. Studies analyzing Caucasian populations in the United States have estimated the incidence to be 146–422 per 100,000 person-years, with an increase of 4%–8% annually.[2,4]

Most BCCs arise from mutations in the hedgehog-signaling pathway. This pathway is of critical importance during embryogenic development as it regulates proliferation, differentiation, and cell fate. Under normal conditions in adults, this pathway is mostly dormant, with the exception of being active in sebaceous glands and hair follicles. Here, hedgehog pathway signaling is responsible for maintaining stem cell population and controlling development. The suppression of this pathway is maintained by patched homolog-1 (PTCH-1) inhibition of smoothened (SMO), the latter being responsible for signal transduction leading to cellular growth in its unsuppressed state. Mutations in the hedgehog pathway leading to tumor growth were discovered during the screening of patients with basal cell nevus syndrome (BCNS, Gorlin syndrome) for hereditary genes. It was initially discovered that a loss of *PTCH-1* suppressor gene function is responsible for this syndrome. Subsequent studies showed this to be the most common mutation (~90% cases) in sporadic BCCs as well. Later, activation mutations in *SMO* were discovered contributing to ~10% cases in sporadic BCCs. Less frequently, a downstream loss of function mutation in the *suppressor of fused gene* (*SUFU*) can also lead to BCC through loss of negative regulation of the hedgehog pathway. Other important mutations found in BCCs include the ultraviolet (UV)-specific *P53* tumor-suppressor gene mutations, which are present in half of BCCs.[2,4,5]

Multiple risk factors contribute to hedgehog pathway mutations and the development of BCC. The most important environmental factor is chronic exposure to UV radiation. Other high-risk factors include fair skin, older age, childhood sunburns, radiation exposure, photosensitizing medications, immune

DOI: 10.1201/9780429026683-3

suppression (iatrogenic or pathologic), arsenic exposure, a family history of skin cancers, tanning bed use, and genetic syndromes predisposing to BCC formation such as Gorlin syndrome and xeroderma pigmentosum.[2,4]

There are multiple clinical and histopathological variants of BCC. The classic appearance of BCC is often used to describe the nodular variant, which typically presents as a thin papule or plaque with raised, rolled, translucent "pearly" borders and overlying telangiectatic vessels, giving a pink hue to the lesion. Under dermoscopy, the vessels have an arborizing appearance, with a milky-pink translucent background. Other subtypes are named based on their clinical appearance or pathological growth pattern. They include superficial BCCs, which tend to present as a red minimally scaly patch or thin plaque mimicking eczema or psoriasis; and pigmented BCCs, which appear as a hyperpigmented brown-black pearly papule. Morpheaform and sclerosing BCCs are variants that could be missed in routine examination as they appear as small atrophic scar-like plaques. Untreated, BCC tends to enlarge slowly, invading deeper tissues, and expanding laterally. Although BCC can enlarge to several centimeters in size, the risk of metastasis continues to be low at 0.0028%–0.5%, with age-adjusted mortality of 0.12 per 100,000.[2–4]

Multiple histological growth patterns have been described in BCC, with more than one pattern occasionally observed in a single tumor. However, all these types share a common histological feature of nests of atypical basaloid cells growing from the epidermis. The nests are characterized by the presence of peripheral palisading, central haphazard arrangement of cells, and clefting (retraction artifact), separating the tumor nests from the surrounding fibromyxoid stroma.[2] The histological growth patterns are divided into low and high risk based on their propensity for recurrence. The main low-risk types include nodular, superficial, and cystic BCCs. High-risk growth patterns include (a) micronodular BCC, characterized by small nests of basaloid cells, and (b) basosquamous BCC, characterized by basaloid cells undergoing squamous differentiation. Another important high-risk histological feature is the presence of perineural invasion, which can be found rarely in any subtype (incidence of <1%).[2–4,6]

Careful assessment of the patient's overall condition is crucial in the management of BCCs. This is true given the various available treatment options, the relatively low risk of BCC recurrence, and rarity of systemic metastasis. The National Comprehensive Cancer Network (NCCN) has updated guidelines for risk assessment, staging, and management of common skin cancers, including BCC. These guidelines are formulated by a consensus among a group of experts who review and summarize the most recent existing data.[7]

Given the slow growth rate, and low risk of BCC metastasis, most therapeutic options target local disease control, which is typically sufficient to achieve complete cure. When choosing a management plan, it is important to keep in mind whether the BCC is of high or low risk for recurrence. The NCCN guidelines divide high-risk factors into clinical and histological factors. The clinical factors associated with high risk of recurrence include any tumor size in high-risk (H) area (central face, eyelids, eyebrows, periorbital, pre/postauricular, nose, lips, chin, mandible, genitalia, hands, and feet); tumor greater than or equal to 1 cm in a medium-risk (M) area (cheeks, forehead, scalp, neck, and pretibial); tumor greater than or equal to 2 cm in a low-risk (L) area (trunk and extremities excluding hands, feet, and pretibial areas); recurrent tumor; previously irradiated areas; immunosuppression; and poorly defined clinical borders. The histological factors associated with high risk of recurrence include perineural invasion and certain histopathologic BCC subtypes (micronodular, infiltrative, basosquamous, and sclerosing/morpheaform types).[3,4,7]

Surgical treatment is the modality most commonly employed to treat BCC. When treating with excision, the NCCN recommends excising with 4 mm clinical margins with post-operative margin assessment for low-risk BCC, and surgical excision with wider margins or Mohs micrographic surgery (MMS) for high-risk BCC.[4,7] MMS is the treatment of choice for high-risk BCC as it offers close to 100% margin assessment. When treating with MMS, the 5-year recurrence rate is 1% for primary tumors and 5.6% for recurrent tumors. This is compared to 10.1% for primary tumors and 17.4% for recurrent tumors when surgical excision is used.[8]

Radiation therapy (RT) has a comparable cure rate to surgical excision and can be used to treat BCC in poor surgical candidates or as an adjuvant therapy for certain high-risk BCCs.[1,9]

Alternative treatments for BCC include electrodessication and curettage (ED&C), cryotherapy, photodynamic therapy (PDT), and topical creams utilizing imiquimod or 5-fluorouracil (5-FU).

These modalities are typically reserved for low-risk, small or superficial BCC and careful patient selection is of high importance. The NCCN recommends ED&C for certain low-risk BCCs, excluding tumors located in terminal hair-bearing areas due to the risk of deep tumor extension along hair follicles.[7] ED&C is considered a cost-effective and quick approach. The main disadvantages of ED&C is that it does not offer margin assessment, is operator-dependent, and tends to heal with worse scarring compared with excision or MMS. The 5-year recurrence rate ranges between 3.3% and 22.7%, depending on the tumor size and location.[4]

PDT is performed utilizing aminolevulinic acid (ALA) or methyl aminolevulinic acid (MAL), and is typically used for patients with multifocal superficial disease or those with extensive background actinic damage. It has a cure rate of 70%–90%. Imiquimod is a cream used once daily, 5 days a week for a total of 6–12 weeks, and has an 81% cure rate. 5-FU is a cream applied twice daily for 3–6 weeks, but treatment may be continued for up to 10–12 weeks if needed.[4] A study found tumor-free survival at 3 years to be 79.7% when using imiquimod, 68.2% with 5-FU, and 58.1% with PDT-MAL.[10] The main disadvantage of topical creams is erythema and excessive irritation which can lead to treatment interruption or poor compliance.[2,4] Systemic therapies are usually reserved for locally advanced BCCs, metastatic BCCs, or for syndromic BCCs (e.g., Gorlin syndrome), and will be discussed further in the case descriptions that follow.

References

1. Garbutcheon-Singh KB, Veness MJ. The role of radiotherapy in the management of non-melanoma skin cancer. *Australas J Dermatol.* 2019;60(4):265–272. doi:10.1111/ajd.13025.
2. Tanese K. Diagnosis and management of basal cell carcinoma. *Curr Treat Options Oncol.* 2019;20(2). doi:10.1007/s11864-019-0610-0.
3. Puig S, Berrocal A. Management of high-risk and advanced basal cell carcinoma. *Clin Transl Oncol.* 2015;17(7):497–503. doi:10.1007/s12094-014-1272-9.
4. Kim DP, Kus KJB, Ruiz E. Basal cell carcinoma review. *Hematol Oncol Clin North Am.* 2019;33(1):13–24. doi:10.1016/j.hoc.2018.09.004.
5. Blanpain C, Fuchs E. Epidermal homeostasis: A balancing act of stem cells in the skin. *Nat Rev Mol Cell Biol.* 2009;10(3):207–217. doi:10.1038/nrm2636.
6. Laurenţiu Mogoantă CLMATB 1 MRMMBIAIPMB. Histological and immunohistochemical study of the eyelid basal cell carcinomas – PubMed: https://pubmed-ncbi-nlm-nih-gov.ezproxy.bu.edu/26429176/. Accessed September 5, 2020.
7. NCCN. National Comprehensive Cancer Network (NCCN). https://www.nccn.org/professionals/physician_gls/pdf/nmsc.pdf. Accessed August 15, 2020.
8. Rowe DE, Carroll RJ, Day CL. Mohs surgery is the treatment of choice for recurrent (previously treated) basal cell carcinoma. *J Dermatol Surg Oncol.* 1989;15(4):424–431. doi:10.1111/j.1524-4725.1989.tb03249.x.
9. Gunaratne DA, Veness MJ. Efficacy of hypofractionated radiotherapy in patients with non-melanoma skin cancer: Results of a systematic review. *J Med Imaging Radiat Oncol.* 2018;62(3):401–411. doi:10.1111/1754-9485.12718.
10. Roozeboom MH, Arits AHMM, Mosterd K, et al. Three-year follow-up results of photodynamic therapy vs. imiquimod vs. fluorouracil for treatment of superficial basal cell carcinoma: A single-blind, noninferiority, randomized controlled trial. *J Invest Dermatol.* 2016;136(8):1568–1574. doi:10.1016/j.jid.2016.03.043.

Case 3.1

Authors: Bilal Fawaz, MD, Sarah Phillips, MD, Sara Al Janahi MD, MSc, Iman Fatima Khan, MS, MPH, and Debjani Sahni, MD.

Reason for Presentation: Management of locally advanced BCC (laBCC).

Chief Complaint: Large ulcer on the right shoulder.

History of Present Illness: An older patient presented to the emergency department (ED) for an acute hemorrhage of an enlarging chronic ulcer on the right upper back that had been present for approximately 15 years. The patient had previously avoided seeking medical help. The patient had declined prior advice for diagnostic studies and had dressed the enlarging ulcer by themselves over the years. After stabilizing the bleeding in the ED, the patient left once again without obtaining a definitive diagnosis or treatment for the ulcer. He again presented to the ED 1 year later with further bleeding from the wound, worsening pain in the right upper extremity, and fatigue.

Review of Systems: Limited range of motion of the right shoulder, with pain in the right arm and shoulder.

Medical/Surgical History: Anemia and type II diabetes mellitus.

Medications: Insulin.

Social History: Nil relevant.

Family History: Nil relevant.

Physical Examination: Right upper back and right shoulder: 14.0 x 13.5 cm ulcer with raised, rolled margins (see Figure 3.1.1).

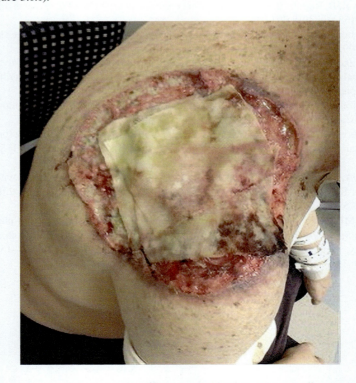

FIGURE 3.1.1 Large, irregular pink ulceration with raised, rolled borders and a non-adherent surgical dressing in the center.

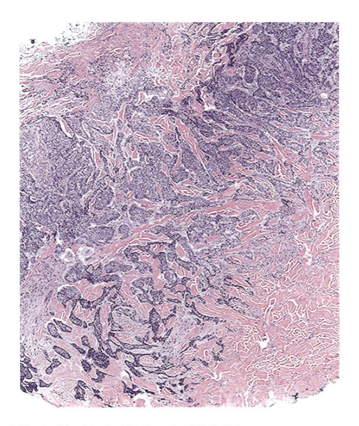

FIGURE 3.1.2 Punch biopsy of the right shoulder ulcer edge (H&E, 40×).

Pathology: Punch biopsy of the right shoulder ulcer edge (see Figure 3.1.2): Narrow strands of basaloid epithelium (H&E, 40×).

Investigations

- **Complete blood count:** Hemoglobin – 6.3 g/dL; hematocrit – 22.2%; mean corpuscular volume (MCV) – 70 FL; platelets – 462 K/μL; white blood cells – 9.1 K/μL; ferritin – 35 ng/mL; iron – 11 mcg/dL; total iron binding capacity (TIBC) – 246.
- **CT right upper extremity with contrast:** An ill-defined area of increased soft tissue density involving the skin and subcutaneous tissues of the posterior right axillary region with extension into the infraspinatus and supraspinatus muscles. Mixed osteolytic/osteosclerotic changes within the scapula and clavicle with new low-density 2.5 cm collection within the subscapularis muscle highly suspicious for abscess. Findings were concerning for chronic osteomyelitis.
- **CT thorax without contrast:** No axillary, mediastinal, or perihilar lymphadenopathy.

Final Diagnosis: laBCC leading to anemia and chronic osteomyelitis of the underlying scapula.

Management and Disease Course: Following the diagnosis of laBCC of the right shoulder and correction of the anemia with transfusion, a wide local excision with grafting was recommended to the patient by surgical oncology. However, the patient refused surgery as he was concerned about limited movement of his right arm following the procedure. Taking the patient's preference into consideration, the option of radiation was discussed in detail together with possible complications from this, including failure to achieve cure, delayed wound healing, and joint contracture. The patient also declined this. Fortunately

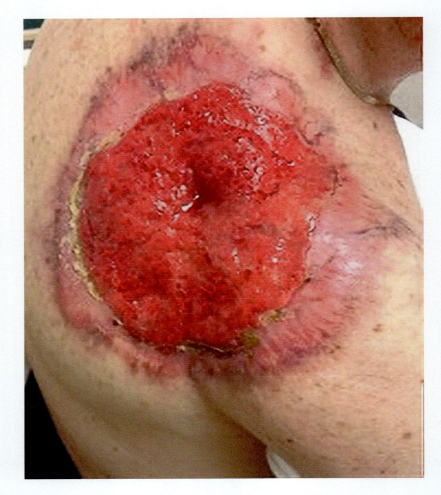

FIGURE 3.1.3 Granulation and resolution of the ulcer with evidence of re-epithelialization at the periphery on the right shoulder.

for the patient, the first hedgehog inhibitor for advanced BCC had just been approved by the FDA and was recommended by the multidisciplinary cutaneous oncology tumor board. The patient agreed to this and vismodegib 150 mg/once daily was started.

The response to vismodegib was remarkable. The ulcer started shrinking visibly within a few weeks of treatment (see Figure 3.1.3) and continued to progressively resolve with scarring (see Figure 3.1.4). Within 8 months of treatment, there was complete resolution of the ulcer with scarring and re-epithelialization. The patient remained systemically well on this therapy but developed side effects of nausea, dysgeusia, and significant hair loss on the scalp. After 10 months of therapy, the patient noticed a new ulceration at the margin of the scar (see Figure 3.1.5). A biopsy from the new ulcer confirmed recurrence of the BCC (see Figure 3.1.6) and emerging drug resistance to vismodegib. A referral was made to radiation oncology to treat the recurrence, but the patient was lost to follow-up.

Discussion

- Vismodegib is the first hedgehog pathway inhibitor to be approved by the FDA for the treatment of metastatic and laBCC.[1–3] The hedgehog signal transduction pathway plays an important role in cellular proliferation and differentiation during embryogenesis.[4] In adults, the pathway

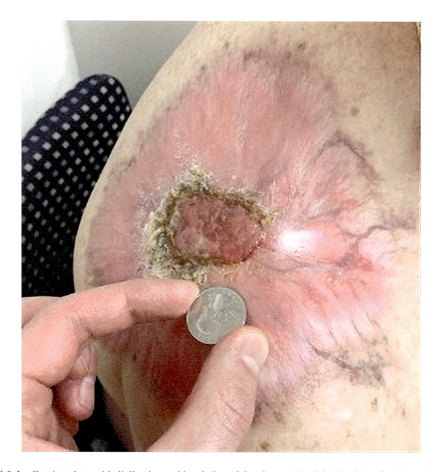

FIGURE 3.1.4 Continued re-epithelialization and involution of the ulcer on the right shoulder after 5 months.

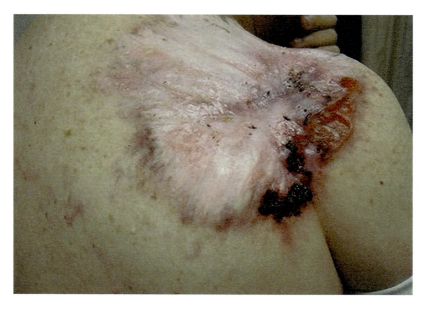

FIGURE 3.1.5 Evidence of ulcer recurrence at the inferolateral margin of the scar on the right shoulder.

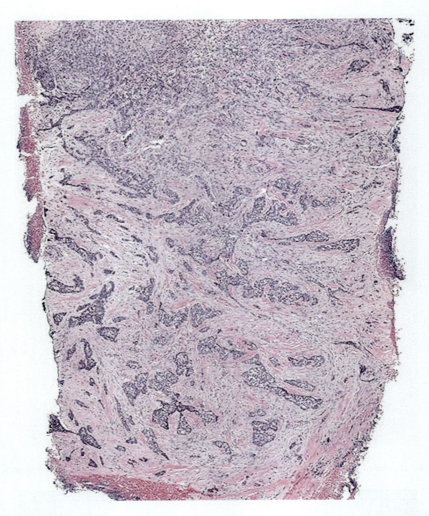

FIGURE 3.1.6 Punch biopsy from the recurrent ulceration on the right shoulder: Infiltrating basaloid epithelium in a desmoplastic myxoid stroma (H&E, 40×).

becomes quiescent in most of the body, outside the skin, hair, and nails.[4] Key regulators within the pathway include the transmembrane receptors patched (PTCH-1) and smoothened (SMO), as well as the hedgehog-signaling ligands Sonic, Indian, and Desert.[4] SMO is the critical activator of the pathway, and PTCH-1 normally suppresses SMO in the absence of the hedgehog ligands, thereby preventing cellular proliferation.[4]

- Ligand binding to PTCH-1 relieves its inhibition of SMO, triggering an intracellular cascade that results in cellular growth via activation of the GLI-1 transcription factor.[4] The inhibition of SMO by PTCH-1 was discovered to be crucial in BCC development as *PTCH-1* mutations are found in 90% of sporadic BCCs.[5] Inactivation of PTCH-1 leads to constitutive activation of SMO, resulting in uninhibited cellular growth and BCC development.[5]

- Vismodegib is a first-in-class, small-molecule, selective inhibitor of SMO, which compensates for the inactivation of PTCH-1 via its direct and potent inhibition of SMO.[1,2] Additionally, vismodegib counteracts activating mutations in SMO, which are present in about 10% of sporadic BCCs.[5]

- Vismodegib has an objective response rate (ORR) of 43.0%–60.3% in laBCC and 30.0%–48.5% in metastatic BCC (mBCC).[1–3] The long-term results of the pivotal ERIVANCE phase II trial included 104 patients, 39 months after accrual.[2] After a median treatment duration of 17.2 months, the ORR was 48.5% in mBCC (all partial responses [PR]) and 60.3% in laBCC (20/38 achieved complete responses [CR] and 18/38 had PRs). The median time to overall response was significantly shorter in mBCC than in laBCC (57 vs. 140 days, respectively), and the 2-year overall survival was lower with mBCC when compared to laBCC (62.3% vs. 85.5%, respectively).[2] Of note, the median duration of response increased from 12.9 to 14.8 months in mBCC and from 7.6 to 26.2 months in laBCC after long-term data evaluation.[1–3]

- Despite the overall positive responses, only 8% of patients remained on vismodegib 39 months post-accrual. Treatment was discontinued in 96/104 patients due to disease progression (27.9%), patient choice (26.0%), and adverse events (21.2%).[2] The most common adverse effects (AEs) are muscle spasms, alopecia, dysgeusia, weight loss, fatigue, and nausea.[1–3] While dysgeusia is not considered to be life-threatening, it commonly leads to drug discontinuation due to its significant impact on patients' quality of life. Vismodegib also has a black box warning regarding the risk of embryofetal death or severe birth defects if given to a pregnant woman. Pregnancy must be ruled out prior to starting vismodegib in females of reproductive potential. Although treatment options for managing AEs from vismodegib are limited, patients should be reassured that the majority resolve by 12 months after discontinuing the drug.[2,3]

- While most patients experience clinical benefit on vismodegib, acquired resistance is common. A retrospective review of 28 patients with advanced BCC demonstrated a resistance rate of 21% after a mean duration of 56.4 weeks.[6] Resistance to vismodegib is secondary to hedgehog pathway reactivation, most commonly involving the drug target SMO.[7] Acquired mutations were found to either interfere with drug binding or directly over-activate SMO.[7] Additionally, mutations involving downstream components of the hedgehog pathway have also been detected, particularly *SUFU* and *GLI-2*.[7]

- Once resistance to vismodegib is encountered, other SMO inhibitors, such as sonidegib, are unlikely to be of clinical benefit. Targeting more downstream effectors in the hedgehog pathway may be more efficacious in overcoming resistance, similar to combination therapy with BRAF and MEK inhibitors in advanced melanoma.[7] Potential agents include BET inhibitors targeting BRD4, which is involved in GLI activation, as well as arsenic trioxide and itraconazole.[8,9] Arsenic trioxide also destabilizes GLI2, inhibiting the hedgehog pathway downstream to SMO, while itraconazole suppresses both SMO and GLI.[9] Clinical studies investigating arsenic trioxide have demonstrated only modest efficacy, but itraconazole has achieved promising results.[9,10] In a phase II, non-randomized clinical trial that included 19 mBCC patients who received itraconazole, the medication resulted in a 24% tumor size reduction and a 65% reduction in hedgehog pathway activity.[10] While further studies are needed, the future of advanced BCC treatment lies in the addition of downstream hedgehog pathway inhibitors to those that directly target SMO.

Teaching Pearls

- Vismodegib, a selective SMO inhibitor, has demonstrated remarkable efficacy in the treatment of metastatic or locally advanced BCC. However, drug resistance and adverse events limit its long-term clinical benefit.
- Common AEs include muscle spasms, alopecia, and dysgeusia.
- Combination therapy with agents targeting downstream hedgehog molecules may help overcome resistance to SMO inhibitors.

References

1. Dessinioti C, Plaka M, Stratigos AJ. Vismodegib for the treatment of basal cell carcinoma: Results and implications of the ERIVANCE BCC trial. *Futur Oncol.* 2014;10(6):927–936. doi:10.2217/fon.14.50.

2. Sekulic A, Migden MR, Basset-Seguin N, et al. Long-term safety and efficacy of vismodegib in patients with advanced basal cell carcinoma: Final update of the pivotal ERIVANCE BCC study. *BMC Cancer.* 2017;17(1). doi:10.1186/s12885-017-3286-5.

3. Sekulic A, Migden MR, Oro AE, et al. Efficacy and safety of vismodegib in advanced basal-cell carcinoma. *N Engl J Med.* 2012;366(23):2171–2179. doi:10.1056/nejmoa1113713.

4. Ingham PW, Nakano Y, Seger C. Mechanisms and functions of Hedgehog signalling across the metazoa. *Nat Rev Genet.* 2011;12(6):393–406. doi:10.1038/nrg2984.

5. Reifenberger J, Wolter M, Knobbe CB, et al. Somatic mutations in the PTCH, SMOH, SUFUH and TP53 genes in sporadic basal cell carcinomas. *Br J Dermatol.* 2005;152(1):43–51. doi:10.1111/j.1365–2133. 2005.06353.x.

6. Chang ALS, Oro AE. Initial assessment of tumor regrowth after vismodegib in advanced basal cell carcinoma. *Arch Dermatol.* 2012;148(11):1324–1325. doi:10.1001/archdermatol.2012.2354.

7. Sharpe HJ, Pau G, Dijkgraaf GJ, et al. Genomic analysis of smoothened inhibitor resistance in basal cell carcinoma. *Cancer Cell.* 2015;27(3):327–341. doi:10.1016/j.ccell.2015.02.001.

8. Long J, Li B, Rodriguez-Blanco J, et al. The BET bromodomain inhibitor I-BET151 acts downstream of smoothened protein to abrogate the growth of hedgehog protein-driven cancers. *J Biol Chem.* 2014;289(51):35494–35502. doi:10.1074/jbc.M114.595348.

9. Cosio T, Di Prete M, Campione E. Arsenic trioxide, itraconazole, all-trans retinoic acid and nicotinamide: A proof of concept for combined treatments with hedgehog inhibitors in advanced basal cell carcinoma. *Biomedicines.* 2020;8(6):156.

10. Kim DJ, Jim J, Spaunhurst K. Open-label, exploratory phase II trial of oral itraconazole for the treatment of basal cell carcinoma. *J Clin Oncol.* 2014;32(8):745–751.

Case 3.2

Authors: Sarah Phillips, MD, Bilal Fawaz, MD, Tatchai Ruangrattanatavorn, MD, MSc, Elizabeth T. Rotrosen, AB, and Adam Lerner, MD.

Reason for Presentation: Treatment approach to metastatic BCC.

Chief Complaint: Non-healing chest wound.

History of Present Illness: An older patient presented with a history of a painful, ulcerating mass on the right chest that had been present over 5 years. The patient had previously refused surgical resection of the mass which had been offered and opted instead for RT at an outside facility. Radiation shrunk the lesion initially, but months after treatment completion, the lesion began to regrow. The patient pursued non-traditional therapies in the interim, including ozone therapy, laser therapy, collagenase cream, hyperbaric oxygen, and activated charcoal, all without effect.

Review of Systems: No pertinent positives.

Medical/Surgical History: Multiple prior BCCs.

Medications: None.

Family History: Nil relevant.

Physical Examination: Right inframammary fold: Large friable ulcerated tumor with raised, rolled borders, moderate drainage, and a fibrinous base (see Figure 3.2.1); Firm, tethered lymphadenopathy of the right axilla was also noted.

Pathology: Punch biopsy of the ulcer edge in the right inframammary fold (see Figure 3.2.2): A nodule of atypical basaloid epithelium in a loose mucinous stroma (H&E, 100×).

Investigation

- **CT chest, abdomen, and pelvis:** 10 × 1.7 cm mass overlying the skin of the right chest. Enlarged lymph nodes in the right axilla measuring 7 × 7 cm and 2.5 cm suspicious for metastatic disease.

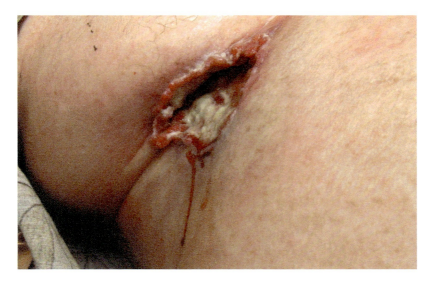

FIGURE 3.2.1 Irregular, deep ulcer with rolled borders in the right inframammary fold.

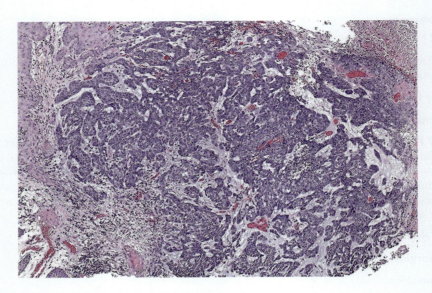

FIGURE 3.2.2   Punch biopsy of the ulcer edge (H&E, 100×).

Final Diagnosis: Metastatic BCC.

Management and Disease Course: The patient declined a diagnostic lymph node aspiration due to their fear and aversion to invasive procedures. Management options for metastatic BCC according to the NCCN guidelines were discussed with the patient, including combinations of surgery, radiation, and hedgehog pathway inhibitors (vismodegib or sonidegib). The patient refused both surgery and radiation, opting instead for vismodegib 150 mg daily. This was despite being informed that treatment with the drug alone was palliative and could not lead to cure as patients ultimately develop drug resistance.

After 3 months of therapy, both the chest and right axillary tumors had decreased in size considerably. This was corroborated by evidence from repeat imaging studies. The patient developed side effects of dysgeusia, mild muscle cramping, and diarrhea; the former two were tolerable, and the latter was alleviated by loperamide. Following the initial significant response, the tumor board advised pulsing the vismodegib with 3 months on followed by 3 months off treatment and then repeating this schedule, in an attempt to stall the development of drug resistance. After gaining confidence through the efficacy of the drug, the patient became more amenable to the idea of surgery and adjuvant radiation. The cutaneous oncology tumor board recommended a debulking surgery of the primary tumor and axillary lymph node dissection after achieving maximum reduction in tumor size from vismodegib. Adjuvant radiation to the tumor and lymph node bed was advised following the debulking surgery, as well as consideration for the off-label use of PD-1 inhibitor therapy. However, after multiple follow-up visits to coordinate this plan, the patient became apprehensive and was subsequently lost to follow-up prior to undergoing the surgery.

Discussion

- LaBCC is defined as a large (>10 mm), recurrent, or aggressive BCC with direct extension into surrounding tissue.[1] The adjusted incidence of laBCC is 226.09 per 100,000 person-years.[1] BCC metastasis occurs in 0.0028%–0.55% of all cases, most commonly in long-standing tumors.[2] Risk factors for metastasis include the head and neck region, male gender, large lesion size, and recurrence following treatment. It typically occurs through lymphatic spread but may also occur hematogenously.[2]

- Vismodegib, a hedgehog pathway inhibitor, has demonstrated remarkable response rates in ~50% of advanced BCC. However, durable responses are limited, and development of resistance is typical, arising within 6–8 months of initiation of therapy. Hedgehog inhibitors should, therefore, not be used as monotherapy for the treatment of advanced BCC with curative intent.[3]

- Given the rarity of presentation of advanced BCC, evidence is limited regarding the best therapeutic approach to achieve durable and effective responses.[4–12] Vismodegib may be used in the neoadjuvant setting prior to more definitive treatment with surgery and/or RT, particularly for laBCC.[4–7] Hedgehog pathway inhibitors result in response rates of 60.3% of laBCC and 48.5% of metastatic BCC. When utilized as neoadjuvant treatment prior to surgery, vismodegib decreased the surgical defect size by 27%.[5] However, one of the main concerns with neoadjuvant vismodegib is the possibility of skip lesion development within areas of resolved tumor. Vismodegib may induce a dormant state in some tumor cells, which subsequently become reactivated following medication discontinuation. As a result, tumor clearance after neoadjuvant vismodegib followed by surgery cannot be truly confirmed until patients have been off treatment for at least 4–6 months.[5]

- Vismodegib may also be combined with RT to potentially improve outcomes in advanced BCC.[6–9] A recent experiment using BCC cell lines demonstrated that vismodegib acts as a radiosensitizer.[6] Specifically, cells treated with vismodegib were more responsive to RT compared to untreated controls due to vismodegib's GLI-1 transcription factor downregulation.[6] In clinical practice, combined use of vismodegib and RT appears to be both safe and effective, although studies so far are limited to case reports.[7–9] A phase II trial is evaluating the safety and tolerability of combined RT and vismodegib (NCT01835626).[10]

- Multiple case reports have also demonstrated benefit in using immunotherapy in advanced BCC. The majority of patients in these reports were treated with PD-1 inhibitors in combination with surgery and/or RT. PD-1 inhibitors are thought to be effective in patients with advanced BCC in part because of their high mutational burden, which is an emerging marker of PD-1 inhibitor effectiveness in the treatment of several cancers.[11] A phase II trial is evaluating the utilization of PD-1 inhibition after progression on hedgehog pathway inhibitors (NCT03132636). Additionally, there is a phase 1b trial evaluating pembrolizumab with or without vismodegib in advanced BCC.[12,13]

Teaching Pearls

- Resistance to vismodegib is inevitable, and hedgehog inhibitors should not be used as monotherapy in the treatment of advanced BCC.
- Vismodegib may be used in the neoadjuvant setting prior to more definitive therapy with surgery and/or radiation to minimize morbidity.
- Vismodegib is a radiosensitizer and has been reported to be used safely and effectively with radiation.
- Immunotherapy with PD-1 inhibitors are currently in trial phase to investigate their use with or after developing resistance to vismodegib.

References

1. Goldenberg G, Karagiannis T, Palmer JB, et al. Incidence and prevalence of basal cell carcinoma (BCC) and locally advanced BCC (LABCC) in a large commercially insured population in the United States: A retrospective cohort study. *J Am Acad Dermatol.* 2016;75(5):957.e2–966.e2.
2. Nikanjam M, Cohen PR, Kato S, et al. Advanced basal cell cancer: Concise review of molecular characteristics and novel targeted and immune therapeutics. *Ann Oncol.* 2018;29(11):2192–2199.
3. Atwood SX, Sarin KY, Whitson RJ, et al. Smoothened variants explain the majority of drug resistance in basal cell carcinoma. *Cancer Cell.* 2015;27(3):342–353.
4. Ally MS, Aasi S, Wysong A, et al. An investigator-initiated open-label clinical trial of vismodegib as a neoadjuvant to surgery for high-risk basal cell carcinoma. *J Am Acad Dermatol.* 2014;71(5):904. e1–911.e1.

 5. Eberl M, Mangelberger D, Swanson JB, et al. Tumor architecture and notch signaling modulate drug response in basal cell carcinoma. *Cancer Cell*. 2018;33(2):229.e4–243.e4.
 6. Hehlgans S, Booms P, Gullulu O, et al. Radiation sensitization of basal cell and head and neck squamous cell carcinoma by the hedgehog pathway inhibitor vismodegib. *Int J Mol Sci*. 2018;19(9):2485. doi: 10.3390/ijms19092485.
 7. Raleigh DR, Algazi A, Arron ST, et al. Induction Hedgehog pathway inhibition followed by combined-modality radiotherapy for basal cell carcinoma. *Br J Dermatol*. 2015;173:544–546.
 8. Pollom EL, Bui TT, Chang AL, et al. Concurrent vismodegib and radiotherapy for recurrent, advanced basal cell carcinoma. *JAMA Dermatol*. 2015; 151:998–1001.
 9. Schulze B, Meissner M, Ghanaati S, et al. Hedgehog pathway inhibitor in combination with radiation therapy for basal cell carcinomas of the head and neck: First clinical experience with vismodegib for locally advanced disease. *Strahlenther Onkol*. 2016;192:25–31.
10. Yom S. *Phase II Study of Radiation Therapy and Vismodegib for Advanced Head/Neck Basal Cell Carcinoma*. Clinical Trial Identifier: NCT01835626.
11. Chen L, Aria AA, Silapunt S, et al. Emerging nonsurgical therapies for locally advanced and metastatic nonmelanoma skin cancer. *Dermatol Surg*. 2019;45(1):1–16.
12. Sanofi. *PD-1 in Patients With Advanced Basal Cell Carcinoma Who Experienced Progression of Disease on Hedgehog Pathway Inhibitor Therapy, or Were Intolerant of Prior Hedgehog Pathway Inhibitor Therapy*. ClinicalTrials.gov Identifier: NCT03132636.
13. Chang A. *Pembrolizumab With or Without Vismodegib in Treating Metastatic or Unresectable Basal Cell Skin Cancer*. ClinicalTrials.gov Identifier: NCT02690948.

Case 3.3

Authors: Sarah Phillips, MD, Malathi Chittireddy, MD, MSc, Hannah E. Mumber, BS, and Bichchau Michelle Nguyen, MD, MPH.

Reason for Presentation: Non-surgical management of BCNS.

Chief Complaint: Multiple skin cancers on the face.

History of Present Illness: The patient presented to a dermatology clinic to discuss management options of six new biopsy-proven BCCs on the face. The patient reported a long history of several BCCs previously treated with surgical excisions, with the first being discovered at age 16. The patient was no longer interested in pursuing further surgery.

Review of Systems: No pertinent positives.

Medical/Surgical History: Severe needle/procedure phobia; BCNS with numerous BCCs treated with either Mohs surgery or excision; excision of multiple prior odontogenic keratocysts and teeth extractions; nasal polyps.

Medications: Nil relevant.

Family History: No family history of skin cancer. No other family members with similar skin cancers.

Social History: Nil relevant.

Physical Examination: Face/neck: Frontal bossing; scattered pink pearly papules with arborizing telangiectasias on the left lateral eyebrow, central forehead, right temple, bilateral cheeks, left nasal sidewall, and left nasal ala (see Figure 3.3.1); Bilateral palms: Multiple, distinct 1–2 mm pits; Back: Sprengel deformity of the right scapula.

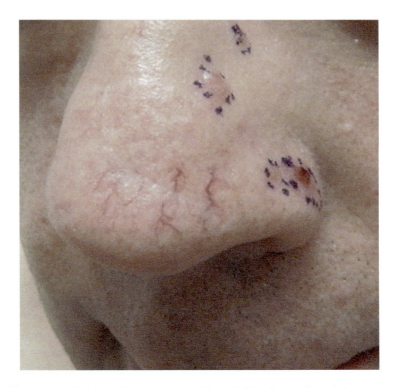

FIGURE 3.3.1 Three scattered pink pearly papules on the left nasal sidewall and left nasal ala.

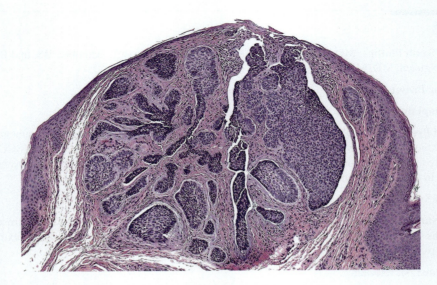

FIGURE 3.3.2   Shave biopsy from the left lateral eyebrow papule (H&E, 100×).

Pathology: Shave biopsy from the left lateral eyebrow papule (see Figure 3.3.2): A well-circumscribed tumor of atypical basaloid epithelium with retraction artifact in a fibromucinous stroma (H&E, 100×); consistent with BCC, nodular type. Additional shave biopsies were taken from the central forehead, right temple, right cheek, left nasal tip, and left cheek also demonstrated BCC, nodular type.

Final Diagnosis: Multiple BCCs in a patient with known BCNS and severe needle/procedure phobia.

Management and Disease Course: Given the presence of multiple BCCs with a background of severe needle phobia, together with the anticipated substantial morbidity from multiple surgeries, oral vismodegib therapy was recommended. Based on unpublished preliminary study data available to us at the time, we advised alternating a 12-week course of vismodegib 150 mg daily with 12 weeks off vismodegib. The patient received PDT once every 4 weeks during the period vismodegib was withheld. This regimen was adopted to limit the undesirable known side effects of vismodegib and allow the patient to tolerate this drug long term. The purpose of PDT was to treat microscopic/dormant BCC and prevent BCC recurrence when vismodegib was withheld.

PDT was administered during the vismodegib "off period" every 4 weeks, utilizing 5-aminolevulinic acid (ALA) and a blue light (400 nm) protocol. The patient was able to complete two courses of alternating vismodegib and PDT therapy (total of 1 year). All BCCs resolved clinically within the first 5 weeks of taking vismodegib. Though some of the BCCs started to recur during the "vismodegib off period", they subsequently resolved later in the treatment course.

Overall, the patient tolerated the medication well. He did develop mild dysgeusia and muscle cramps while on vismodegib, but these side effects resolved completely during the 12 weeks vismodegib was held. At the end of the year, the patient was noted to have complete clinical response with no evidence of any recurrent or clinically suspicious new BCCs (see Figure 3.3.3). He was very satisfied with his response but was then lost to follow-up.

Discussion

- BCNS, also called Gorlin's syndrome, is a challenging condition for dermatologists to manage due to the large number of BCCs that patients often accumulate. There is no gold standard approach to treating multiple BCCs in the setting of BCNS. The treatment options available for patients with BCNS who present with multiple BCCs are essentially the same as those available to treat a solitary BCC in a patient without BCNS.

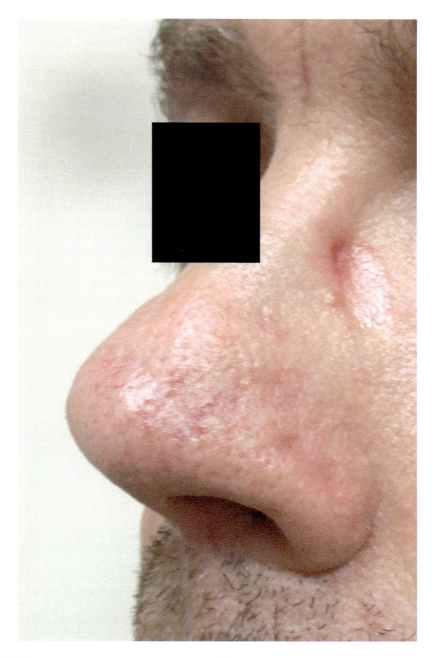

FIGURE 3.3.3 Post-treatment atrophic scars on the left nasal sidewall and left nasal ala.

- Vismodegib, a hedgehog pathway inhibitor, approved for the treatment of locally advanced and metastatic BCC, has also been shown to be effective for patients with BCNS. A double-blind randomized controlled trial revealed that patients with BCNS receiving 150 mg vismodegib daily developed significantly fewer new BCCs per year relative to patients on placebo (a mean of 2 vs. 34 new surgically eligible BCCs per year, respectively $P<0.0001$). The study demonstrated the long-term safety of vismodegib (up to 36 months) with excellent disease control and without developing drug resistance. However, only 13% of the patients in the study who received vismodegib were able to tolerate the drug continuously without a treatment break due to side effects. These were most commonly muscle cramps, hair loss, and dysgeusia. Stopping the drug also led to disease recurrence, even though at the time of drug cessation there had appeared to be both clinical and histological disease resolution. When the drug was restarted there was a return of clinical benefit as well as adverse events.[1]

- It is interesting to note that vismodegib is effective not only for multiple BCCs in patients with BCNS but also for the odontogenic keratocysts that these patients commonly develop.[2] This is likely due to the shared genetic pathophysiology underlying these conditions, specifically related to mutations in the *PTCH1* gene.[3]
- Another randomized double-blind, multi-center trial demonstrated the safety and efficacy of two different intermittent dosing regimens for vismodegib. One group was treated with vismodegib 150 mg daily for 12 weeks, followed by three courses of placebo (8 weeks) alternating with vismodegib 12 weeks. The second group was treated with vismodegib 150 mg daily for 24 weeks, followed by three courses of placebo (8 weeks) alternating with vismodegib (8 weeks). Both treatment regimens demonstrated efficacy, which was not affected by treatment interruption. The alternating regimens led to better long-term tolerability of vismodegib.[4]
- In addition to counseling patients with BCNS on treatment options for existing BCCs, providers must also counsel patients on prevention strategies to mitigate the risk of future BCCs. These include advising strict sun protection, limiting diagnostic radiation, and considering nicotinamide supplementation at a dose of 500 mg twice daily.[5]

Teaching Pearls

- Vismodegib may be used to reduce morbidity, both physical and psychological, associated with undergoing numerous surgical procedures for patients presenting with multiple BCCs such as in BCNS.
- Intermittent dosing with vismodegib provides an alternative treatment strategy in patients presenting with multiple BCCs in terms of safety and efficacy, while enabling better tolerability of the drug when taken long term.

References

1. Tang JY, Ally MS, Chanana AM, et al. Inhibition of the hedgehog pathway in patients with basal-cell nevus syndrome: Final results from the multicentre, randomised, double-blind, placebo-controlled, phase 2 trial. *Lancet Oncol.* 2016;17(12):1720–1731.
2. Booms P, Harth M, Sader R, et al. Vismodegib hedgehog-signaling inhibition and treatment of basal cell carcinomas as well as keratocystic odontogenic tumors in Gorlin syndrome. *Ann Maxillofac Surg.* 2015;5(1):14–9. doi:10.4103/2231–0746.161049.
3. Akbari M, Chen H, Guo G, et al. Basal cell nevus syndrome (Gorlin syndrome): Genetic insights, diagnostic challenges, and unmet milestones. *Pathophysiology.* 2018;25(2):77–82. doi:10.1016/j.pathophys.2017.12.004.
4. Dréno B, Kunstfeld R, Hauschild A, et al. Two intermittent vismodegib dosing regimens in patients with multiple basal-cell carcinomas (MIKIE): A randomised, regimen-controlled, double-blind, phase 2 trial. *Lancet Oncol.* 2017;18(3):404–412.
5. Chen AC, Martin AJ, Choy B, et al. A phase 3 randomized trial of nicotinamide for skin-cancer chemoprevention. *N Engl J Med.* 2015;373(17):1618–1626.

Case 3.4

Authors: Bilal Fawaz, MD, Hannah Kopelman, DO, and Michael A. Dyer, MD.

Reason for Presentation: Definitive treatment of a nasal BCC with radiation.

Chief Complaint: Non-healing ulcer on the nose.

History of Present Illness: An elderly patient presented with a 2-year history of an enlarging painful, ulcerated lesion on the left nasal ala which bled intermittently. After being lost to follow-up for a year following the initial presentation, the patient presented to the dermatology clinic a second time.

Review of Systems: Negative.

Medical/Surgical History: Previously had a BCC excised from the back, hypertension, congestive heart failure, chronic kidney disease, poorly controlled psychiatric illness.

Medications: Aspirin, levothyroxine, metolazone, potassium chloride, metoprolol succinate, torsemide.

Allergies: Chlordiazepoxide, potassium nitrate.

Family History: No family history of skin cancer.

Social History: Issues with permanent housing.

Physical Examination (at initial presentation): A 2 cm shallow ulcer with hemorrhagic base and rolled, pearly borders on the left nasal ala.

Pathology: Punch biopsy, left nasal ala ulcer: Narrow strands of atypical basaloid cells infiltrating the dermis, consistent with BCC, infiltrative type.

Physical Examination (1 year after initial visit): A 3.5 cm well-defined ulcer with scant fibrinous debris, central hemorrhagic crust, and raised rolled borders, involving the left nasal sidewall, ala, with extension onto the left medial cheek and infraorbital region (see Figure 3.4.1); no palpable cervical, axillary, or inguinal lymphadenopathy.

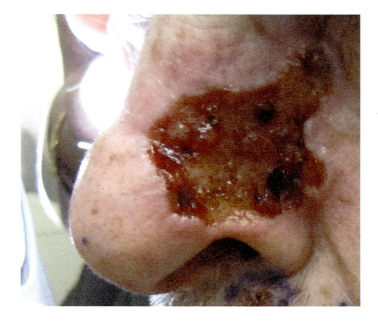

FIGURE 3.4.1 Large, irregular, centrally ulcerated plaque with raised rolled borders involving the left nasal ala, sidewall, and left infraorbital region.

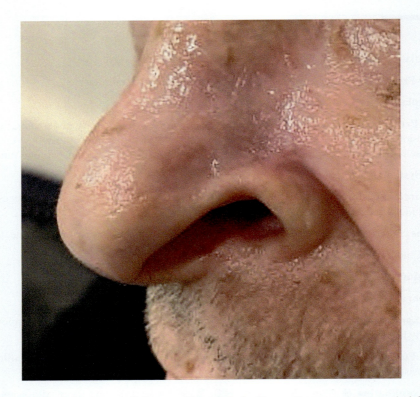

FIGURE 3.4.2   Well-healed scar post-radiotherapy with no clinical evidence of tumor persistence on the left nose.

Management: Mohs surgery with reconstruction was advised, given its large size and high-risk location. However, the patient failed to attend several scheduled appointments for surgical management because of underlying poorly controlled psychiatric illness and homelessness. After returning to the clinic a year later with worsening pain, increased bleeding, and enlargement of the ulcer to 3.5 cm, the lesion now extended from the nasal ala, up the nasal side wall, and toward the left lower eyelid (see Figure 3.4.1). The patient declined surgery but did agree to RT.

The patient underwent CT simulation for three-dimensional RT planning. The patient was treated with electron external-beam radiotherapy using 9 MeV electrons, receiving 66 Gy in 33 fractions at 2 Gy per fraction over 6.5 weeks (with daily treatments from Monday to Friday). A custom metal block was used to shape the radiation beam, and an external eye shield was placed for protection over the left eye at every treatment. A daily 1 cm bolus was used to ensure adequate dose at the skin surface.

The patient tolerated RT well with the expected side effects of radiation dermatitis (managed with petrolatum) and moist desquamation (managed with silver sulfadiazine) in the treatment field. There was significant regression of the lesion and resolution of symptoms during treatment. One month after RT, the moist desquamation had resolved, and the ulcer was no longer visible, with an excellent cosmetic result (see Figure 3.4.2).

Discussion

- Treatment options for facial BCCs include surgery (Mohs surgery or wide local excision with frozen section control of the surgical margins), definitive radiotherapy, or systemic therapy (e.g., hedgehog pathway inhibitors such as vismodegib).[1]
- Fortunately, most BCCs are slow growing and have a high cure rate with surgery alone, and they rarely metastasize. The 5-year cause-specific survival for a localized BCC is 99%, with

rates of regional lymph node metastasis as low as 0.1%.[2] However, untreated BCCs can cause extensive damage via local invasion. Tumors associated with a worse prognosis include those with poorly defined borders, perineural invasion, or aggressive histopathology, for example, sclerosing, basosquamous, and morpheaform BCC types.[2]

- Radiotherapy is a valuable tool in the management of BCCs and can be used as an adjuvant treatment, particularly in cases of positive margins (where resection is not feasible or functionally not desirable), significant perineural invasion, bone invasion, or recurrent disease. Radiotherapy can also be used as a definitive primary treatment option in place of surgery, particularly in patients of advanced age who may not wish to undergo surgery, or in those with multiple comorbidities where surgery can pose a significant risk.[3] NCCN guidelines recommend that RT be offered to non-surgical candidates and patients over 60 years of age.[4] RT can be a particularly useful treatment modality for tumors in sensitive locations, where surgery could pose a risk to important functions of the face or poor cosmetic outcome. Radiation treatment can allow preservation of the structure and the function of the eyelid, nasal ala, nasal tip, and lip.[5]

- There is only one randomized trial comparing local control rate in cases of definitive RT with definitive surgery for BCCs. The study showed a 4-year actuarial local control rate of 92.5% for RT compared with 99.3% for surgery ($P=0.003$). Four-year patient-reported cosmesis was also better in the surgery arm.[6] However, this trial used what are now considered outdated radiation techniques, including absence of CT simulation for three-dimensional treatment planning.[6] Contemporary definitive RT for BCC is associated with 5-year local control rates of approximately 95%.[4]

- Different RT modalities may be utilized for the treatment of BCCs: (a) Electron-beam RT; (b) surface brachytherapy (either electronic, or high-dose rate radioisotope); and (c) superficial orthovoltage X-rays. All three allow for deposition of the radiation dose superficially, with much less dose deposited deeper into the body, which is ideal for most skin cancers. Locally advanced, unresectable BCCs, or those with positive lymph nodes or extensive perineural invasion, may be treated with another modality called (d) intensity-modulated radiation therapy (IMRT), which involves photon beams entering the body from multiple different angles. Each beam is partially blocked from every angle to create a dose distribution conforming to the unique shape of the target (e.g., the tumor, the lymph node basin, or the course of a nerve) while simultaneously sparing the critical surrounding normal tissues from the high-dose radiation. In more recent times, patients with advanced BCC can also be treated with hedgehog pathway inhibitors as neoadjuvant treatment prior to using radiation.

- Both electron-beam radiation therapy and IMRT are types of *external*-beam radiation therapy that rely on the creation of high-energy (i.e., megaelectron-voltage) electrons or photons by a large machine called a linear accelerator. The electron setting of linear accelerators is commonly used instead of the photon setting to treat BCCs because electrons are less penetrating. Different energy electrons (e.g. 6 versus 9 versus 12 MeV) are associated with different surface doses and different depths of penetration, and the radiation oncologist can use different energy electrons, custom blocks, internal or external eye shields, and "bolus", that is, any substance placed on the skin to increase radiation dose at the surface to create the ideal radiation dose distribution for a given patient.

- In contrast to external-beam radiation, surface brachytherapy uses a radioactive source placed in close proximity to the skin via an "applicator" (e.g., a flexible flap containing a series of catheters). High-dose rate radioisotope surface brachytherapy, in particular, can create a more even dose distribution on curved surfaces compared to electron external-beam radiation. While surface brachytherapy is increasingly utilized to treat skin cancers, it is not considered standard radiation treatment in the 2020 NCCN guidelines and should only be delivered at specialized radiation oncology facilities in carefully selected patients.[4]

- One of the challenging aspects of RT from patients' perspectives is multiple clinic visits per week for several weeks. Typical RT doses for definitive treatment of BCCs and SCCs are

60–70 Gy in 30–35 fractions (2 Gy per fraction) over 6–7 weeks. Treatments are generally short (i.e., less than 20 minutes), and acute side effects, most commonly mild fatigue, as well as radiation dermatitis and alopecia in the treatment area, build up slowly over the course of treatment. Acute radiation dermatitis is typically managed topically, with a combination of emollients and mid-to-low potency topical corticosteroids, depending on the site. If ulceration is present, absorbent dressings are recommended to protect against contamination, control pain, and absorb secretions. The most common long-term side effect is permanent alopecia in the treatment field, but atrophy, dyspigmentation, and telangiectasias can also occur, frequently many years after treatment. Hypofractionated radiotherapy, that is, the delivery of RT over a shorter number of sessions by delivering a higher dose per fraction, is associated with equivalent local control, but worse long-term cosmetic outcomes.[5] Acceptable hypofractionated schedules include 40 Gy in 10 fractions over 2 weeks and 30 Gy in five fractions over 2–3 weeks.[4] However, traditionally fractionated regimens are generally preferred for larger tumors, those involving bone or cartilage, or when cosmesis is a high priority. Cosmetic outcomes are generally good or excellent with standard fractionated RT.[5]

Teaching Pearls

- Choosing the appropriate treatment for a patient with BCC depends on patient-specific factors such as age, social and psychiatric status, and patient values and preference, patient comorbidities, as well as disease factors, such as tumor size, depth, histopathology, and location.
- RT is an effective and generally very well tolerated definitive treatment option for BCC, especially in patients of advanced age or those who are poor surgical candidates due to comorbidities. The decision to use definitive RT for a particular BCC is best made by radiation oncologists in conjunction with dermatologists and individual patients.
- Various RT modalities and treatment schedules can be used to treat BCC, with more protracted schedules associated with better long-term cosmetic outcomes. A radiation oncologist's decision regarding what modality and treatment schedule to use will depend on the availability of the different modalities, the patient's goals and values, and the anatomic, clinical, and histopathologic characteristics of the BCC to be treated.

References

1. Rubin AI, Chen EH, Ratner D. Current concepts: Basal-cell carcinoma. *N Engl J Med*. 2005;353(21): 2262–2269.
2. Mierzwa ML. Radiotherapy for skin cancers of the face, head, and neck. *Facial Plast Surg Clin North Am*. 27(1):131–138.
3. Strom TJ, Harrison LB. Radiotherapy for management of basal and squamous cell carcinoma. *Curr Probl Cancer*. 2015;39(4):237–247.
4. National Comprehensive Cancer Network. Basal Cell Skin Cancer (Version 1.2020). https://www.nccn.org/professionals/physician_gls/pdf/nmsc_blocks.pdf. Accessed April 26, 2020.
5. Strom TJ, Caudell JJ, Harrison LB. Management of BCC and SCC of the head and neck. *Cancer Control*. 2016;23(3): 220–227.
6. Avril MF, Auperin A, Margulis A, et al. Basal cell carcinoma of the face: Surgery or radiotherapy? Results of a randomized study. *Br J Cancer*. 1996;76 (1):100–106.

4

Cutaneous Lymphoma

Bilal Fawaz and Debjani Sahni

CONTENTS

Overview

Cutaneous lymphomas are a diverse group of lymphoproliferative disorders with a wide range of clinical presentations, histologic findings, and prognoses.[1–6] An important initial distinction is whether the neoplasm develops primarily in the skin (i.e., primary cutaneous lymphoma [PCL]), or if it represents secondary involvement of the skin by a systemic lymphoma.[1] PCLs have a better prognosis compared to secondary cutaneous disease from a systemic lymphoma (5-year survival of approximately 90% vs. 31%, respectively).[7]

The overall annual incidence of PCL is approximately 10.0 per million person-years, accounting for 19% of extranodal lymphomas.[3] PCLs are subdivided into cutaneous T-cell lymphoma (CTCL), cutaneous B-cell lymphoma (CBCL), and other lymphomas arising from natural killer (NK) cells.[3] CTCL is the most common subtype, accounting for 65% of all PCLs, with an estimated incidence of 6.4 per million person-years.[3] CBCL is the second most common subtype of PCL, accounting for ~25% of cases.[1,2] Due to disease heterogeneity, each subtype of PCL is further subdivided into various disease categories based on a combination of clinical findings, histologic features, and/or molecular analyses.

Cutaneous T-Cell Lymphoma

CTCL is classified into three main categories: (a) Classic CTCL (65%), which includes mycosis fungoides (MF) and Sézary syndrome (SS); (b) primary CD30+ lymphoproliferative disorders (25%), which include cutaneous anaplastic large-cell lymphoma (C-ALCL) and lymphomatoid papulosis (LyP); and (c) other CTCL (10%), which encompasses a group of often aggressive lymphomas, such as subcutaneous panniculitis-like T-cell lymphoma, extranodal NK/T-cell lymphoma nasal type, and cutaneous

DOI: 10.1201/9780429026683-4

peripheral T-cell lymphoma, not otherwise specified.[1–3] Men are almost twice as likely to develop CTCL than women, and incidence among blacks is higher than other racial groups.[3] The disease presents at a median age of 55–60 years, but certain variants differ significantly in their age of onset (e.g., hypopigmented MF predominately presents in the pediatric population).[3]

MF represents the most common form of CTCL overall, with an annual incidence of 0.4/100,000 in the United States.[3] This generally indolent lymphoma is characterized by a protracted evolution of disease stage from patch to plaque, and eventually to tumor stage, often requiring years to progress between the stages. Additionally, not all patients progress to more advanced stages, and may remain, for example, as patch stage for the rest of their life.[5,6] Diagnosis is often delayed due to the considerable variability in clinical presentation, often mimicking benign skin disorders, and because non-specific histologic findings are typically seen early in the disease process.[5]

Clinically, MF initially develops as irregular, erythematous patches with fine overlying scale and variable degrees of atrophy, telangiectasia, and pigmentary changes.[5] The patches may slowly progress to indurated plaques and eventually to tumors in a minority of patients (~10%). However, patients do not develop more advanced lesions such as tumors without first having gone through the earlier stages of patch and plaque. Therefore, should a patient present with tumor lesions only with no prior patches or plaques, the diagnosis will ultimately be a CTCL *other* than MF.[5,6] The "bathing suit" distribution with a predilection for the buttocks, inguinal region, thighs, and lower abdomen is a characteristic distribution of MF in its early stages.[5] Several clinical variants of MF exist, including poikilodermatous MF (formerly known as poikiloderma vasculare atrophicans), hypopigmented MF, folliculotropic MF, pagetoid reticulosis, and granulomatous slack skin.[5]

The histologic findings vary according to stage, but key features include a lichenoid lymphocytic infiltrate with epidermotropism and dermal sclerosis.[1,5,6] Diagnosing MF can often be elusive as biopsies are often non-diagnostic, especially early in the disease course.[1,5,6] Adequate tissue sampling is of utmost importance in maximizing a diagnosis of MF being made, often necessitating multiple and/or larger biopsy specimens from different lesions. If both patch and plaque lesions are present, the biopsy is more likely to yield a diagnostic result if the sample is taken from a plaque. Biopsies should be avoided, where possible, from tumor lesions as epidermotropism is often lost in tumors. It is also helpful to have the skin biopsy specimen undergo technical preparation by cutting along the long axis of the specimen rather than the usual "bread loafing". Immunophenotyping and T-cell gene rearrangement studies serve as adjunctive studies that may aid in confirming the diagnosis. However, even with molecular studies, the final result may not be diagnostic, and clinicopathologic correlation is therefore essential in making a final diagnosis of CTCL.[1,5,6]

The staging of MF and SS was developed and published in 1979 by the Mycosis Fungoides Cooperative Group (MFCG) and is based on tumor-node-metastasis classification. In 2007 this was revised and updated by the International Society for Cutaneous Lymphoma (ISCL) and the cutaneous lymphoma task force of the European Organization of Research and Treatment of Cancer (EORTC). The purpose was to incorporate more recent advances and molecular data in CTCL into the staging system. In particular the incorporation of blood involvement (B) which is an important prognostic variable in patients with MF and SS (Table 4.1).[4] Skin-directed therapies are the preferred treatment of choice in the early stages of MF.[5] Topical corticosteroids, topical nitrogen mustard, topical bexarotene, phototherapy (psoralen plus ultraviolet A [PUVA], NBUVB), and radiotherapy are most often used.[5] For patients who require systemic therapy, oral bexarotene, interferon-alpha, and low-dose methotrexate and extracorporeal photopheresis are often considered lower down the treatment ladder. Other therapeutic options for more advanced disease include alemtuzumab, mogamulizumab, romidepsin, and brentuximab vedotin along with various chemotherapeutic agents, including cyclophosphamide, liposomal doxorubicin, and pralatrexate.[5]

The prognosis in MF patients is favorable, with an overall disease-specific survival of 89% and 75% at 5 and 10 years, respectively.[5,6] However, outcomes differ significantly between stages. Patients with patch/plaque-stage MF have an excellent prognosis, with a 5-year disease-specific survival of 100% and 96% for stages IA and IB, respectively.[5,6] In contrast, patients with stage III disease have a 40% 5-year disease-specific survival.[5] Therefore, close monitoring of all MF patients is essential to regularly update staging and tailor treatment accordingly.

TABLE 4.1

ISCL/EORTC Revision to the Classification of Mycosis Fungoides and Sézary Syndrome

TNMB Stages

Skin

T1 Limited patches,[a] papules, and/or plaques[b] covering <10% of the skin surface. May further stratify into T1a (patch only) vs T1b (plaque ± patch)

T2 Patches, papules, or plaques covering ≥10% of the skin surface. May further stratify into T2a (patch only) vs T2b (plaque ± patch)

T3 One or more tumors[c] (≥1 cm diameter)

T4 Confluence of erythema covering ≥80% body surface area

Node

N0 No clinically abnormal peripheral lymph nodes[d]; biopsy not required

N1 Clinically abnormal peripheral lymph nodes; histopathology Dutch grade 1 or NCI N0–2

N1a Clone negative[g]

N1b Clone positive[g]

N2 Clinically abnormal peripheral lymph nodes; histopathology Dutch grade 2 or NCI LN3

N2a Clone negative[g]

N2b Clone positive[g]

N3 Clinically abnormal peripheral lymph nodes; histopathology Dutch grades 3–4 or NCI LN4; clone positive or negative

Nx Clinically abnormal peripheral lymph nodes; no histologic confirmation

Visceral

M0 No visceral organ involvement

M1 Visceral involvement (must have pathology confirmation[e] and organ involved should be specified)

Blood

B0 Absence of significant blood involvement: ≤5% of peripheral blood lymphocytes are atypical (Sézary) cells[f]

B0a Clone negative[g]

B0b Clone positive[g]

B1 Low blood tumor burden: >5% of peripheral blood lymphocytes are atypical (Sézary) cells but does not meet the criteria of B2

B1a Clone negative[g]

B1b Clone positive[g]

B2 High blood tumor burden: ≥1,000/µL Sézary cells[f] with positive clone[g]

Source: From Ref. [4] with permission.

a For skin, patch indicates any size skin lesion without significant elevation or induration. Presence/absence of hypo- or hyperpigmentation, scale, crusting, and/or poikiloderma should be noted.

b For skin, plaque indicates any size skin lesion that is elevated or indurated. Presence or absence of scale, crusting, and/or poikiloderma should be noted. Histologic features such as folliculotropism or large-cell transformation (>25% large cells), CD30+ or CD30−, and clinical features such as ulceration are important to document.

c For skin, tumor indicates at least one 1 cm diameter solid or nodular lesion with evidence of depth and/or vertical growth. Note total number of lesions, total volume of lesions, largest size lesion, and region of body involved. Also note if histologic evidence of large-cell transformation has occurred. Phenotyping for CD30 is encouraged.

d For node, abnormal peripheral lymph node(s) indicates any palpable peripheral node that on physical examination is firm, irregular, clustered, fixed or 1.5 cm or larger in diameter. Node groups examined on physical examination include cervical, supraclavicular, epitrochlear, axillary, and inguinal. Central nodes, which are not generally amenable to pathologic assessment, are not currently considered in the nodal classification unless used to establish N3 histopathologically.

e For viscera, spleen and liver may be diagnosed by imaging criteria.

f For blood, Sézary cells are defined as lymphocytes with hyperconvoluted cerebriform nuclei. If Sézary cells are not able to be used to determine tumor burden for B2, then one of the following modified ISCL criteria along with a positive clonal rearrangement of the TCR may be used instead: (a) Expanded CD4+ or CD3+ cells with CD4/CD8 ratio of 10 or more, (b) expanded CD4+ cells with abnormal immunophenotype including loss of CD7 or CD26.

g A T-cell clone is defined by PCR or Southern blot analysis of the T-cell receptor gene.

SS accounts for less than 5% of all CTCL and occurs exclusively in adults.[4,8] While it was initially thought to be a leukemic MF variant, recent studies have demonstrated that SS and MF may be distinct disorders arising from separate T-cell subsets.[8] SS is characterized by the triad of erythroderma, generalized lymphadenopathy, and the presence of peripheral Sézary T-cells.[8] The disease often presents with severely pruritic, exfoliative, erythematous patches and plaques, encompassing >80%–90% of the body surface area (BSA).[1,8] Because it is often challenging to distinguish SS from other causes of erythroderma, certain criteria are required to confirm the diagnosis, including: (a) Absolute Sézary cell count >1,000 cells/μL *or* CD4+/CD8+ ratio >10 *or* aberrant expression of pan-T-cell antigens; *and* (b) T-cell clonality in the peripheral blood.[1,8] The prognosis of SS is poor, with past studies documenting an overall 5-year survival of 25%, often due to secondary opportunistic infections; however, survival may be improving with the availability of modern therapy.[8]

CD30-positive cutaneous neoplasms are the second most common group of CTCL, representing ~25% of cases.[1–3] This group encompasses a wide spectrum of disorders, including primary cutaneous lymphoproliferative disorders (LyP and PC-ALCL), CD30+ transformed MF, systemic ALCL with secondary cutaneous involvement, and other CTCL that may express CD30.[1] The conditions are difficult to distinguish based on histology alone as they often have overlapping histologic and immunophenotypical features. Therefore, clinicopathologic correlation is crucial in establishing the correct diagnosis.[1]

PC-ALCL accounts for 12% of all CTCLs, most often arising in adults with a male:female ratio of 2:1.[1–3] The disease presents with solitary (80%) or multifocal (20%) nodules and tumors, often with secondary ulceration.[1] Lesions are characterized by partial or complete spontaneous regression with a high rate of relapse.[1] A diffuse dermal infiltrate of large, atypical CD4+ lymphocytes is present on histopathology, and at least 75% of the cells should express CD30 to confirm the diagnosis.[1] Overall, 10% of the patients develop extracutaneous disease involving regional nodes, though prognosis remains favorable as the 10-year overall survival is >85%.[1,2] Due to the localized nature of the disease, skin-directed therapies are often first line, most commonly radiotherapy or surgical excision.[1]

LyP exists on a spectrum with PC-ALCL and is characterized by a chronic, waxing and waning course.[1–3] It accounts for 15% of CTCLs and can occur at any age.[3] Clinically, LyP is characterized by the presence of small, red-brown, centrally crusted or necrotic papules in various stages of evolution.[1] Hypo or hyperpigmented macules and varioliform scars may also be present. The eruption is generally asymptomatic and has a predilection for the trunk and extremities.[1] Establishing the diagnosis is essential given the association of LyP with an additional malignancy in up to 20% of cases. The second malignancy most commonly being MF, PC-ALCL, or Hodgkin's lymphoma.[1] Despite this association, the prognosis of LyP remains favorable overall.[1] First-line therapies include topical corticosteroids, phototherapy with or without interferon-alpha, retinoids, and methotrexate.[1]

Cutaneous B-Cell Lymphoma

CBCLs represent ~25% of all cutaneous lymphomas and are classified into three main types: Primary cutaneous marginal zone lymphoma (PCMZL), primary cutaneous follicle center lymphoma (PCFCL), and primary cutaneous diffuse large B-cell lymphoma, leg-type (PC-DLBCL).[1] PCFCL and PCMZL are low-grade, indolent malignancies with an overall good prognosis, whereas PC-DLBCL is known to behave more aggressively and have a worse overall survival rate.[1] For all CBCLs, it is essential to perform a thorough staging evaluation at the time of diagnosis to rule out secondary cutaneous involvement by a systemic B-cell lymphoma as the prognosis is worse and the approach to treatment is very different in the latter scenario. Investigations include a CBC, CMP, LDH, flow cytometry of peripheral blood, CT of the chest, abdomen, pelvis, and, if feasible/indicated, PET/CT.[1]

PCFCL is the most common subtype of CBCL, mainly affecting adults with a median age of 51 years.[1] This malignancy is characterized by disorganized growth of germinal center cells, leading to pink-violaceous nodules, tumors, or plaques with surrounding erythema, usually on the scalp, forehead, and back.[1] Patients are generally asymptomatic and do not have accompanying B symptoms, such as fevers, chills, or night sweats.[1] Histologically, a diffuse or nodular lymphocytic infiltrate is present, and immunohistochemical staining allows its distinction from other forms of cutaneous lymphomas. All CBCLs are positive for CD-20, which is a well-established B-cell marker.[1] PCFCL is also positive for Bcl-6 and negative for Bcl-2 and MUM-1, enabling its distinction from other CBCLs.[1] While recurrence may occur in up to 50% of patients, systemic dissemination is uncommon, and prognosis is overall favorable.[1]

PCMZL falls within the category of extranodal mucosa-associated lymphoid tissue (MALT) lymphomas according to the WHO classification.[4] Patients present with pink-brown-violaceous papules, plaques, and nodules favoring the upper extremities, lower extremities, and trunk.[1] Lesions often do not ulcerate. Similar to PCFCL, patients are generally asymptomatic, and the prognosis overall is excellent, with a 5-year survival rate of almost 100%.[1] Histologically, PCMZL also presents with a nodular or diffuse dermal infiltrate. Positive staining for CD20, CD79a, and Bcl-2 coupled with negative staining for Bcl-6 and MUM-1 helps to confirm the diagnosis.[1]

For both PCFCL and PCMZL, treatment varies depending on the extent of involvement. Localized disease responds well to topical/intralesional steroids, surgical excision, and radiotherapy, while systemic therapy in the form of rituximab may be used for more extensive disease.[1]

PC-DLBCL, leg-type occurs almost exclusively in elderly women.[1] As the name implies, this lymphoma arises commonly on the distal legs. However, the same designation still applies in 20% of cases involving other body sites, most notably the upper extremities and trunk.[1] H&E findings are similar to other forms of CBCL, but IHC staining is positive for Bcl-2, MUM-1, FOX-P1, and MYC. Bcl-6 staining is variable and not helpful in establishing the diagnosis.[1] In contrast to the first two CBCLs, extracutaneous disease is common, and prognosis is less favorable, with a disease-specific 5-year survival of only 40%–50%.[1] Systemic chemotherapy with R-CHOP is often recommended, with or without adjuvant radiotherapy.[1]

References

1. Sokołowska-Wojdyło M, Olek-Hrab K, Ruckemann-Dziurdzińska K. Primary cutaneous lymphomas: diagnosis and treatment. *Postep Derm Alergol*. 2015;5:368–383.
2. Willemze R, Jaffe ES, Burg G, et al. WHO-EORTC classification for cutaneous lymphomas. *Blood*. 2005;105:3768–3785.
3. Criscione VD, Weinstock MA. Incidence of cutaneous T-cell lymphoma in the United States, 1973–2002. *Arch Dermatol*. 2007;143:854–859.
4. Olsen E, Vonderheid E, Pimpinelli N, et al. Revisions to the staging and classification of mycosis fungoides and Sezary syndrome: a proposal of the International Society for Cutaneous Lymphomas (ISCL) and the Cutaneous Lymphoma Task Force of the European Organization of Research and Treatment of Cancer (EORTC). *Blood*. 2007;110:1713–1722.
5. Kim YH, Liu HL, S Mraz-Gernhard, et al. Long-term outcome of 525 patients with mycosis fungoides and Sezary syndrome: clinical prognostic factors and risk for disease progression. *Arch Dermatol*. 2003;139:857–866.
6. Abbott R, Sahni D, Robson A, et al. Poikilodermatous mycosis fungoides: a study of its clinicopathological, immunophenotypic, and prognostic features. *J Am Acad Dermatol*. 2011;65(2):313–319.
7. Lee WJ, Won KH, Won CH. Secondary cutaneous lymphoma: comparative clinical features and survival outcome analysis of 106 cases according to lymphoma cell lineage. *Br J Dermatol*. 2015;173:134–145.
8. Campbell JJ, Clark RA, Watanabe R, et al. Sezary syndrome and mycosis fungoides arise from distinct T-cell subsets: a biologic rationale for their distinct clinical behaviors. *Blood*. 2010;116:767–771.

Case 4.1

Authors: Elizabeth T. Rotrosen, AB, Bilal Fawaz, MD, and Debjani Sahni, MD.

Reason for Presentation: Successful therapy with brentuximab vedotin in tumor stage MF.

Chief Complaint: Development of large bumps with a background of known MF.

History of Present Illness: An older patient presented in 2006 (then aged 52) for evaluation of a rash which was diagnosed as stage IB MF at an outside institute. Therapy with PUVA was initiated, but the patient was referred to our care after progressing on this therapy. Initially, oral bexarotene was started, but after developing tumor lesions of MF, therapy was switched to liposomal doxorubicin which controlled his disease for the next 10 years with minimal side effects. A lapse in therapy occurred between 2018 and 2020 due to insurance issues, resulting in the patient developing multiple progressive ulcerating painful nodules with associated extreme pruritus.

Review of Systems: Positive for mild fatigue; no pertinent positives otherwise.

Medical/Surgical History: None.

Medications: None.

Family History: Nil relevant.

Social History: Former smoker.

Physical Examination: Fitzpatrick skin type V; Confluent hyperpigmented scaly plaques across the neck, back, and extremities bilaterally (Figure 4.1.1). Several ulcerating papules and nodules with excoriation; small palpable bilateral inguinal adenopathy <1.5 cm diameter.

Pathology: Repeat biopsy was deferred given established diagnosis of MF; initial punch biopsy from the right arm (2006): Perifollicular lymphocytic infiltrate with admixed eosinophils and mucin deposition within the follicular epithelium, confirmed via positive colloidal iron staining, suggestive of folliculotropic mycosis fungoides. Immunoperoxidase staining revealed CD3 (+), CD4 (+), CD8 (−), and CD30 (−) lymphocytes within the epidermis.

Investigations

- **PET-CT whole body:** Multiple cutaneous and subcutaneous nodules bilaterally on the legs and thighs with mild FDG avidity (metabolic activity) involving the right inguinal nodes.
- HTLV-1 negative.

Final Diagnosis: Tumor stage folliculotropic mycosis fungoides (FMF) (stage IIB).

Management and Disease Course: In 2020, the patient addressed his insurance issues and re-established care at our institute. Liposomal doxorubicin was re-initiated given its prior success, but on this occasion, there was no response. The cutaneous oncology tumor board recommendation was to switch to brentuximab vedotin. Skin improvement was noted within one week of the first infusion. The nodules began to heal, bleeding stopped, and the pruritus improved markedly. The patient's skin cleared after four cycles of therapy following which treatment was stopped. There has been no disease recurrence so far after 2 years of follow-up.

Discussion

- MF is the most common subtype of CTCL, accounting for 50%–65% of CTCL cases.[1] Studies have shown that 1%–2% of patients with stage IA or IB MF at diagnosis progress to stage IIB (tumor stage).[2] Patients with stage IIA MF at diagnosis (as in the case of our patient) have a

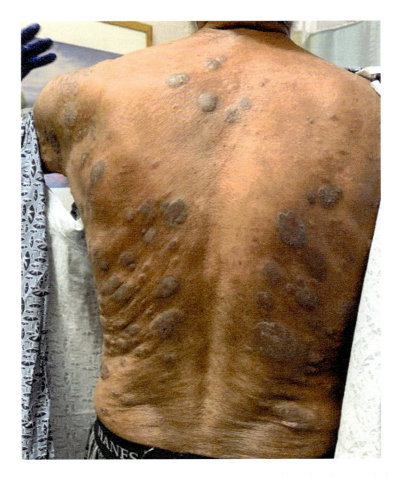

FIGURE 4.1.1   Numerous hyperpigmented-violaceous scaly plaques symmetrically distributed on the back.

higher risk of disease progression (up to 9.4%).[2] Advanced stage at presentation, elevated LDH, and folliculotropic MF are independent predictors of an increased risk of disease progression.[3,4]

- MF is not curable, but treatment leads to long-term responses in the majority of patients. When skin-directed therapies fail, various systemic treatments have demonstrated efficacy in the treatment of MF, including oral bexarotene, methotrexate, liposomal doxorubicin, pralatrexate, and brentuximab vedotin.[5,6]

- Brentuximab vedotin is an anti-CD30 antibody-drug conjugate whose mechanism of action is explained in more detail in Case 4.6.[7,8] Although brentuximab targets the CD30 receptor, its efficacy is not always predictable by the CD30 positivity of the tumor. This is in part due to the unreliability of immunohistochemistry (IHC) staining for CD30. The cutoffs for CD30 positivity are not standardized, and the interpretation of the staining pattern varies considerably between pathologists. In a three-round reproducibility assessment of CD30 staining among 15 pathologists and resident pathologists, agreement of CD30 positivity by IHC was as low as 26%.[9]

- Additionally, a meta-analysis of five clinical trials, three of which included MF patients, demonstrated that CD30 positivity was not predictive of response to brentuximab. The ALCANZA study included 50 patients with MF, of whom 28 showed at least 10% CD30 expression, and 22 exhibited CD30 expression less than 10%. Overall, 71% of participants with CD30 expression ≥10% showed a response to brentuximab compared to 55% of participants with <10% CD30 positivity.

In 35-IST-001, 20 participants showed CD30 expression ≥10% and 20 had <10% CD30 expression. In this study, response to brentuximab was 55% for both levels of CD30 expression. In the 35-IST-002 study, 12/15 participants (80%) with ≥10% CD30 expression showed a positive response to brentuximab treatment compared with 9/17 (53%) of participants with <10% CD30 expression.[10] A separate report on the ALCANZA study showed that higher levels of CD30 expression at baseline were predictors of treatment response to brentuximab, but also observed meaningful responses to treatment with brentuximab in participants with lower levels of CD30 expression.[11]

- The ALCANZA study was a multicenter international, open-label, randomized, phase 3 trial of brentuximab versus physicians' choice (bexarotene or methotrexate) in 131 patients with CD30-positive CTCL (either MF or PC-ALCL).[12] The primary outcome measure of the study was the percentage of participants achieving an objective response rate (ORR) lasting at least 4 months. The ORR to brentuximab was 56.3% versus 12.5% to physicians' choice drug. Complete response (CR) was observed in 17.2% of participants receiving brentuximab treatment versus 1.6% of participants receiving methotrexate or bexarotene. The median duration of progression-free survival was 16.7 months in the brentuximab treatment group compared to 3.5 months in the physicians' choice group.[12] Side effects of brentuximab are discussed in more detail in Case 4.6.

Teaching Pearls

- Brentuximab is an effective treatment for tumor stage MF, even in cases of tumors expressing low levels of CD30.
- The response is relatively quick and durable with an intravenous dosing schedule every 3 weeks which many patients prefer compared to the regimens of other systemic therapies.

References

1. Amorim GM, Niemeyer-Corbellini JP, Quintella DC, et al. Clinical and epidemiological profile of patients with early stage mycosis fungoides. *Anais Brasileiros de Dermatol.* 2018;93:546–552.
2. Quaglino P, Pimpinelli N, Berti E, et al. Time course, clinical pathways, and long-term hazards risk trends of disease progression in patients with classic mycosis fungoides. *Cancer.* 2012;118:5830–5890.
3. Agar NS, Wedgeworth E, Crichton S, et al. Survival outcomes and prognostic factors in mycosis fungoides/ Sézary syndrome: validation of the revised International Society for Cutaneous Lymphomas/European Organisation for Research and Treatment of Cancer Staging proposal. *J Clin Oncol.* 2010;28:4730–4739.
4. Talpur R, Singh L, Daulat S, et al. Long-term outcomes of 1,263 patients with mycosis fungoides and sézary syndrome from 1982 to 2009. *Clin Cancer Res.* 2012;18:5051–5060.
5. Zackheim HS, Kashani-Sabet M, McMillan A. Low-dose methotrexate to treat mycosis fungoides: a retrospective study in 69 patients. *J Am Acad Dermatol.* 2003;49:873–878.
6. Olek-Hrab K, Maj J, Chmielowska E, et al. Methotrexate in the treatment of mycosis fungoides—a multicenter observational study in 79 patients. *Eur Rev Med Pharmacol Sci.* 2018;22:3586–3594.
7. Van De Donk NWCJ, Dhimolea E. Brentuximab vedotin. *MAbs.* 2012;4:458–465.
8. Mehra T, Ikenberg K, Moos RM, et al. Brentuximab as a treatment for CD30+mycosis fungoides and sézary syndrome. *JAMA Dermatol* 2015;151:73.
9. Koens L, Van De Ven PM, Hijmering NJ, et al. Interobserver variation in CD30 immunohisto-chemistry interpretation; consequences for patient selection for targeted treatment. *Histopathology.* 2018;73:473–482.
10. Jagadeesh D, Horwitz SM, Bartlett NL, et al. Response to brentuximab vedotin by CD30 expression: results from five trials in PTCL, CTCL, and B-cell lymphomas. *J Clin Oncol.* 2019;37:7543.
11. Kim YH, Prince HM, Whittaker S, et al. Superior clinical benefit of brentuximab vedotin in mycosis fungoides versus physician's choice irrespective of CD30 level or large cell transformation status in the phase 3 ALCANZA study. *Blood.* 2018;132:1646.
12. Prince HM, Kim YH, Horwitz SM, et al. Brentuximab vedotin or physician's choice in CD30-positive cutaneous T-cell lymphoma (ALCANZA): an international, open-label, randomised, phase 3, multicen-tre trial. *Lancet.* 2017;390:555–566.

Case 4.2

Authors: Bilal Fawaz, MD, Nicole Patzelt, MD, Malathi Chittireddy, MD, MSc, Hannah E. Mumber, BS, and Adam Lerner, MD.

Reason for Presentation: Refractory SS treated with romidepsin.

Chief Complaint: Widespread rash.

History of Present Illness: An elderly patient presented with a 3-year history of a widespread rash associated with pruritus that was significantly affecting his quality of life and disturbing his sleep at night. The patient's primary care provider initially believed it was a drug eruption, but the symptoms did not improve despite discontinuing several medications, resulting in referral to dermatology for evaluation and management.

Review of Systems: Ten-pound weight loss in 3 months.

Past Medical/Surgical History: Asthma, type II diabetes mellitus, hypertension, and hypercholesterolemia.

Medications: Aspirin, hydroxyzine, rosiglitazone, and atorvastatin.

Family History: No family history of skin cancer.

Physical Examination: Erythroderma with leonine facies (Figure 4.2.1); No palmoplantar keratoderma was observed; Small palpable bilateral inguinal lymphadenopathy <1.5 cm diameter.

Pathology: Incisional biopsy of a plaque on the back (Figure 4.2.2): (A) Epidermis showing lymphocytic epidermotropism arranged as single cells and scattered Pautrier microabscesses (H&E, 200×); (B) the majority of tumor cells are positive with immunoperoxidase staining for CD4 (200×); and (C) only a few cells are positive for CD8 (200×).

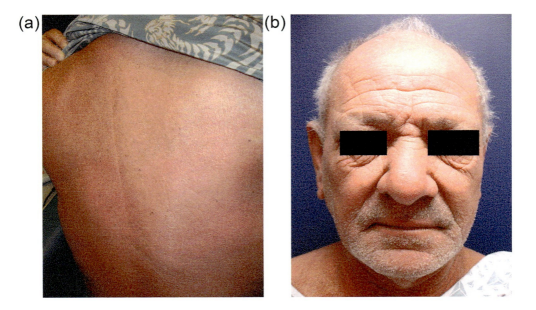

FIGURE 4.2.1 (a) Confluent scaly erythematous patches along the back and (b) deeply furrowed indurated plaques with background erythema on the face.

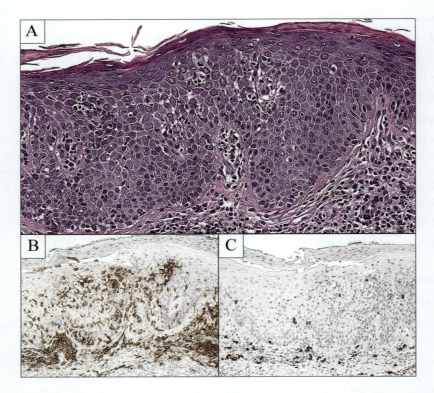

FIGURE 4.2.2   Incisional biopsy from a plaque on the back: (A) H&E, 200×; (B) CD4 immunoperoxidase staining; and (C) CD8 immunoperoxidase staining.

Investigations

Sézary Flow Cytometry:
- CD4: 71%, CD4 (absolute): $1,764/mm^3$
- CD8: 14%, CD8 (absolute): $352/mm^3$
- CD4:CD8 ratio 5:1
- CD4 POS/CD7 negative: 5% CD4 POS/CD7 negative (absolute): $292/mm^3$
- CD4 POS/CD26 negative: 83% CD4 POS/CD26 negative (absolute): $4,852/mm^3$
- Clonality in blood: Positive for TCR (T-cell gene rearrangement)

Final Diagnosis: SS (T4N0M0B2; stage IVA1).

Management and Disease Course: Over the course of 8 months, the patient failed multiple systemic treatments, including oral bexarotene with extracorporeal photopheresis and interferon-alpha-IIB, chlorambucil, alemtuzumab, and pralatrexate. Iatrogenic hypertriglyceridemia prevented the use of higher doses of oral bexarotene. Although he had a good clinical response to pralatrexate, the treatment had to be discontinued due to severe mucositis. As a result, the cutaneous oncology tumor board team recommended initiating treatment with romidepsin 14 mg/m^2 IV on days 1, 8, and 15 of a 28-day cycle.

The patient had an excellent response to romidepsin after 15 months of therapy, with complete clearance of his skin disease and blood involvement (Figure 4.2.3). He developed mild thrombocytopenia and lymphopenia, which did not require any intervention. The patient was gradually transitioned from romidepsin to photopheresis for maintenance therapy, and he continued to have no evidence of recurrence after 13 treatments, so photopheresis was subsequently discontinued. The patient remains in remission off treatment now for 5 years.

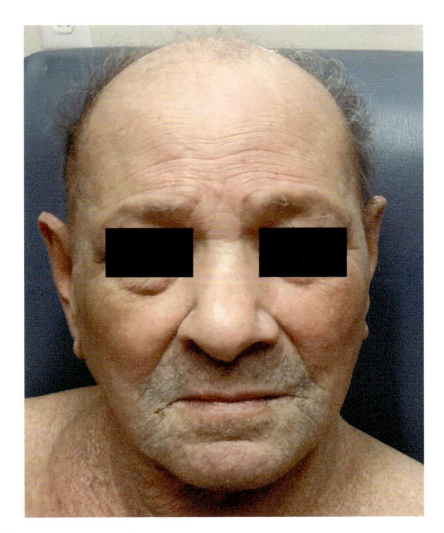

FIGURE 4.2.3 Resolution of leonine facies and erythroderma.

Discussion

- For CTCL patients with advanced disease, a combination of skin-directed and systemic therapy is often required.[1] Numerous agents have reported efficacy in CTCL, including oral retinoids, methotrexate, chlorambucil, and pralatrexate, among others.[1] In patients with refractory disease, histone deacetylase (HDAC) inhibitors, such as romidepsin, may be considered.[1–3]

- Romidepsin is a class 1-specific HDAC inhibitor that is FDA-approved for patients with CTCL who have received at least one prior systemic treatment.[2] HDAC normally functions to block transcription via de-acetylation of DNA.[3] HDAC inhibition prevents the removal of acetyl groups, thereby allowing DNA to remain transcriptionally active. HDAC inhibitors reverse abnormal epigenetic states associated with multiple malignancies, via activation of genes involved in tumor suppression, cell cycle arrest, and apoptosis.[3]

- Romidepsin, in particular, has demonstrated rapid and durable responses in multiple phase II trials, even though most patients had advanced disease and were heavily pretreated with at least one systemic agent.[4,5] In the pivotal Whittaker trial, 96 patients with CTCL were included, with the majority (71%) having stage IIB disease or higher.[4] Six patients (6%) experienced a CR and 27 (28%) experienced a partial response (PR), with an overall response rate of 34%.[2] The median duration of response was 15 months, and the median time to CR was 4.4 months.[2] The trial also demonstrated a clinically meaningful reduction in pruritus in 43% of their patients.[4]

- The Piekarz trial reported similar outcomes in 71 patients with CTCL.[5] CR was noted in four patients (6%), and PR was noted in 30% of the patients, with an ORR of 35%.[5] The responses were also reported to be durable and rapid as the median duration of response was 11 months and the median time to CR was 7.5 months.[3]

- Romedepsin is overall well-tolerated.[4,5] The most common adverse events include vomiting, nausea, fatigue, infection, and transient thrombocytopenia and neutropenia. In the two trials discussed earlier, 21% and 11% of patients experienced treatment discontinuation due to adverse events, and two patients experienced sudden cardiac deaths.[4,5] A subsequent study evaluating the rate of cardiac events with romidepsin found mild QTc interval changes that were clinically insignificant.[6] Because hypokalemia and hypomagnesemia can result from antiemetics, chemotherapy, or the underlying disease, it is recommended that electrolyte levels are monitored and repleted prior to and during treatment with romidepsin.[4–6]

- Romidepsin is primarily metabolized by the cytochrome P-450 isoenzyme 3A4.[2] Other drugs that are known inducers or inhibitors of this system should be avoided during romidepsin treatment. It also binds estrogen receptors and can reduce the efficacy of estrogen-containing contraceptives. As with many medications, its effects have not been specifically investigated in pregnant women, but fetal risk is assumed, and romidepsin should be avoided in pregnancy.[2]

Teaching Pearls

- Romidepsin, a class 1-specific HDAC inhibitor, has demonstrated rapid and durable responses in patients with refractory CTCL.
- Romidepsin has a favorable safety profile with the most common adverse events being nausea, vomiting, loss of appetite, mild thrombocytopenia, and neutropenia.
- Electrolytes should be repleted prior to and during romidepsin therapy.

References

1. Photiou L, van der Weyden C, McCormack C, et al. Systemic treatment options for advanced-stage mycosis fungoides and sézary syndrome. *Curr Oncol Rep.* 2018;20(4):32. doi:10.1007/s11912-018-0678-x.
2. McGraw A. Romidepsin for the treatment of T-cell lymphomas. *Am J Health Syst Pharm.* 2013;70(13):1115–1122.
3. Nakajima H, Kim YB, Terano H, et al. FR901228, a potent antitumor antibiotic, is a novel histone deacetylase inhibitor. *Exp Cell Res.* 1998; 241:126–133.
4. Whittaker S, Demierre M, Kim E, et al. Final results from a multicenter, international pivotal study of romidepsin in refractory cutaneous T-cell lymphoma. *J Clin Oncol.* 2010;28(29):4485–4491.
5. Piekarz R, Frye R, Turner M, et al. Phase II multi-institutional trial of the histone deacetylase inhibitor romidepsin as monotherapy for patients with cutaneous T-cell lymphoma. *J Clin Oncol.* 2009;27(32):5410–5417.
6. Cabell C, Bates S, Piekarz R, et al. Systematic assessment of potential cardiac effects of the novel histone deacetylase (HDAC) inhibitor romidepsin. *Blood.* 2009;114:3709.

Case 4.3

Authors: Sarah Ann Kam, MD, Tatchai Ruangrattanatavorn, MD, MSc, Elizabeth T. Rotrosen, AB, and Michael A. Dyer, MD.

Reason for Presentation: FMF with successful response to low-dose total skin electron beam radiation.

Chief Complaint: Multiple skin lesions on face, trunk, arms, and legs.

History of Present Illness: A middle-aged patient presented with a 12-year history of stage IIB FMF for which multiple forms of therapy were attempted with mixed PRs. Treatments included both skin-directed (topical corticosteroids, topical imiquimod, topical bexarotene, and phototherapy using broadband-UVB and PUVA) and systemic therapies (pralatrexate, romidepsin, brentuximab vedotin, and liposomal doxorubicin). The treatments, though initially helpful, ultimately failed to provide a durable response. Some treatments could not be tolerated due to severe side effects (e.g., brentuximab vedotin induced severe pneumonitis). The treatment at time of presentation was pegylated liposomal doxorubicin, which provided a satisfactory partial response for almost 10 years. More recently, there was widespread gradual worsening of skin lesions consistent with disease progression.

Review of Systems: None.

Medical/Surgical History: Hypertriglyceridemia; history of stage IA malignant melanoma s/p wide local excision.

Medications: Atorvastatin.

Physical Examination: Large scaly plaque above an area of alopecia on the posterior scalp; Multiple coalescing scaly papules and plaques on the neck and chest (Figure 4.3.1); Perifollicular, grouped papules on the upper back with scattered papules on the upper extremities and large annular plaques on the thighs bilaterally; No palpable cervical, axillary, or inguinal lymphadenopathy.

Pathology: Punch biopsy of a plaque on the left upper back (Figure 4.3.2): (a) A superficial and mid-dermal perivascular and interstitial lymphocytic infiltrate; (b) exocytosis of variably sized lymphocytes

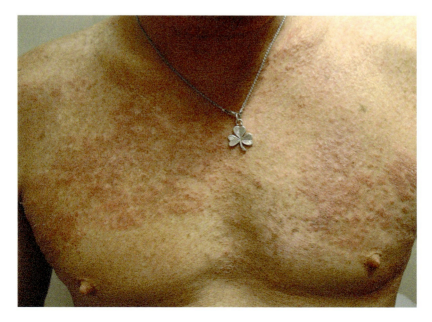

FIGURE 4.3.1   Irregular pink, scaly papules coalescing into larger plaques on the chest bilaterally.

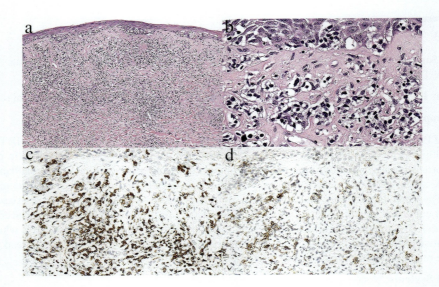

FIGURE 4.3.2   Punch biopsy of a plaque on the left upper back: (a) H&E, 20×; (b) H&E, 300×; (c) positive CD3 immunoperoxidase stain (200×); and (d) positive CD30 immunoperoxidase stain (200×).

with hyperchromatic nuclei in the epidermis and dermis and papillary dermal fibrosis; (c) immunoperoxidase staining with CD3 highlights the epidermotropic and dermal lymphocytes; and (d) immunoperoxidase staining with CD30 reveals positive scattered large lymphocytes consistent with large-cell transformation.

Final Diagnosis: Progression of known FMF.

Management and Disease Course: Treatment options for patients with MF stage IIB include skin-directed therapies and systemic therapies. This was a challenging case of FMF resistant to multiple prior treatment modalities. Given the positive data for radiation use in FMF, low-dose total skin electron beam therapy (TSEBT), 12 Gy in 12 fractions over 3 weeks was initiated. After completing radiation treatment, there was near-complete resolution of all the lesions. During treatment, the patient experienced hair loss and hand swelling which resolved after a month.

A year later, the patient's disease relapsed, prompting a referral for allogeneic stem cell transplantation. Another course of low-dose TSEBT was given which led to rapid disease control. The TSEBT enabled bridging between systemic therapy and transplant enabling the patient to enter into a successful transplantation while under disease remission.

Discussion

- FMF is a rare, aggressive variant of MF that is often associated with a worse prognosis compared to classic MF. Similarly, it is typically less responsive to traditional treatments used for classic MF. More recently, studies have demonstrated the existence of a subgroup of FMF that can behave in a more indolent manner with excellent prognosis.[1] FMF is heterogeneous in the morphology of its rash. Lesions range from comedonal and acneiform papules, keratosis pilaris-like, and follicular-centric papules, in addition to patches, plaques, and tumors, as seen in classic MF. FMF most commonly presents in the head and neck area with associated alopecia, although trunk and extremity lesions also occur.[2]

- It has been suggested that FMF could be classified into three subgroups based on the clinicopathologic presentation that have been shown to demonstrate variable survival rates (see Table 4.2).[1]

TABLE 4.2

Folliculotropic Mycosis Fungoides Classification

Clinical Subgroup	Histopathology	5-Year Overall Survival	10-Year Overall Survival
Early-stage cutaneous disease limited to follicular-based papules or thin plaques	Sparse perifollicular and intrafollicular infiltrates	92	72
Advanced-stage cutaneous disease presenting as thick, infiltrated plaques, tumors, nodules, erythroderma	Diffuse infiltrates containing many medium- to large-sized atypical T-cells	55	28
FMF with extracutaneous spread	–	23	2

Source: Adapted from data in Ref. [1].

- Patients classified as early stage typically respond to less aggressive skin-directed treatments (SDT) such as potent topical steroids and phototherapy. In general, PUVA appears to be more effective than narrowband UVB. In patients with advanced-stage FMF, the above treatments are less effective, and radiotherapy (local radiotherapy and total skin electron beam therapy) has been shown to be the most efficacious.[1–3] Solitary plaques/tumors of MF can be treated with definitive local radiation therapy, 24–30 Gy, usually in 2 Gy per fraction. Patients with more extensive disease, but with limited sites that are progressive or particularly symptomatic, can be treated with a palliative course of localized radiation therapy, 8–12 Gy in 1–3 fractions. In patients with widespread disease, TSEBT is an option.

- TSEBT is a technically challenging form of radiotherapy that can be delivered to patients with advanced cutaneous disease and requires significant physics and dosimetry support. As with other forms of electron beam radiotherapy, TSEBT is delivered via a linear accelerator. However, with TSEBT, advanced techniques are used to administer electron radiation to the entire surface of the skin. Most radiation oncology departments do not have a TSEBT program, and patients should be treated at centers with sufficient experience with this technique. Standard dosing of TSEBT is 30–36 Gy delivered over a period of 8–10 weeks. This dosing, however, is associated with significant skin toxicity, including dermatitis, desquamation, blistering, alopecia, and nail loss. Repeat treatment is usually not given due to cumulative radiation toxicity.[4]

- More recently, groups have recommended low-dose TSEBT (10–12 Gy delivered over a period of 3 weeks) for advanced-stage MF. Individual lesions can be boosted to higher doses, as indicated. Low-dose TSEBT has been shown to have high response rates, with CR in 27% (and in three of eight, or 37.5% of FMF patients specifically) and CR or PR in 88% of patients in one pooled analysis.[3] This is admittedly lower than the 59% CR and 100% CR or PR rates associated with standard-dose TSEBT.[1] However, even with standard dosing, durable complete responses are rare.[1] Because MF is considered a chronic, incurable disease, low-dose TSEBT is generally favored over standard-dose TSEBT as it can be administered multiple times with reduced toxicity compared to higher doses.[3,4]

- Of note, in high-risk, treatment-refractory MF patients, TSEBT can be used to "bridge" patients progressing on systemic therapies to allogeneic stem cell transplantation. The use of TSEBT under these circumstances enhances the likelihood that such patients enter their transplant process with a more durable remission, thereby preventing recurrence while awaiting stem cell engraftment.

Teaching Pearls

- FMF is a rare variant of MF which may be grouped into early-stage FMF, advanced-stage FMF, and extracutaneous FMF based on the clinicopathological presentation and prognosis.

- Whereas less aggressive skin-directed therapy can be effective in early-stage FMF, this is typically not the case for advanced-stage FMF. In the latter, radiation therapy can be very effective as monotherapy or in combination with other therapies such as PUVA.
- TSEBT is an effective treatment in patients with widespread disease. The disadvantages are associated skin toxicity, long duration of treatment, and inability to repeat treatment in the case of disease relapse due to cumulative radiation toxicity. In recent years, low-dose TSEBT has gained more favor due to shorter, better tolerated treatments and the ability to retreat in cases of disease relapse.

References

1. van Santen S, van Doorn R, Neelis KJ, et al. Recommendations for treatment in folliculotropic mycosis fungoides: report of the Dutch Cutaneous Lymphoma Group. *Br J Dermatol.* 2017;177(1):223–228. doi:10.1111/bjd.15355.
2. Muniesa C, Estrach T, Pujol RM, et al. Folliculotropic mycosis fungoides: clinicopathological features and outcome in a series of 20 cases. *J Am Acad Dermatol.* 2010;62(3):418–426. doi:10.1016/j.jaad.2009.03.014.
3. Hoppe RT, Harrison C, Tavallaee M, et al. Low-dose total skin electron beam therapy as an effective modality to reduce disease burden in patients with mycosis fungoides: results of a pooled analysis from 3 phase-II clinical trials. *J Am Acad Dermatol.* 2015;72(2):286–292. doi:10.1016/j.jaad.2014.10.014.
4. Chowdhary M, Song A, Zaorsky NG, et al. Total skin electron beam therapy in mycosis fungoides-a shift towards lower dose? *Chin Clin Oncol.* 2019;8(1):9. doi:10.21037/cco.2018.09.02.

Case 4.4

Authors: Shawn Shih, MD, Bilal Fawaz, MD, and Debjani Sahni, MD.

Reason for Presentation: Successful treatment of poikilodermatous MF with phototherapy.

Chief Complaint: Rash all over body.

History of Present Illness: A young patient presented with a 5-year history of an asymptomatic, generalized rash. The eruption first appeared on the left hip and then spread quickly to cover most of the body. The patient was previously evaluated by multiple dermatologists and had been diagnosed with pityriasis rosea, vasculitis, and, most recently, pigmented purpuric dermatosis. The patient had tried topical steroids, intralesional corticosteroids, and laser treatments, all of which helped a little but did not lead to resolution of the rash.

Review of Systems: No pertinent positives.

Medical/Surgical History: None.

Medications: Doxycycline 100 mg once daily (for acne vulgaris).

Family History: Second degree relative with non-Hodgkin's lymphoma.

Social History: Nil relevant.

Physical Examination: Skin type III; Lower abdomen, upper and lower extremities, flanks, back: Moderately defined erythematous-brown patches with background of telangiectasia and focal areas of hypopigmentation within the patches (Figure 4.4.1); the lesions on the extremities appeared less poikilodermatous, especially anteromedially on the thighs with moderately defined, large, red-brown patches with overlying fine scale and wrinkling; Face: Few scattered erythematous papules on cheeks and temporal areas bilaterally; Body surface area (BSA) ~50%–60%; No palpable lymph nodes.

Pathology: Shave biopsy from the right hip: Atypical lymphocytes, focally in clusters, tagging the dermoepidermal junction, band-like lymphocytic infiltrate, dermal fibrosis, and scattered pigment laden macrophages; shave biopsy from the abdomen: The population of atypical lymphocytes tagging the dermoepidermal junction is CD3 (+), CD8 (+) over CD4 (+), and partial loss of CD7 and CD5.

Investigations

- CBC and CMP within normal limits
- Antinuclear antibody screen negative

Final Diagnosis: Poikilodermatous MF, stage 1B (T2aN0M0B0).

Management and Disease Course: No further diagnostic studies were pursued because the patient's disease was early stage. Doxycycline was discontinued, and the patient was scheduled for phototherapy (nbUVB) three times per week given the large BSA of involvement and prior literature on poikilodermatous MF. After 15 months of phototherapy at a frequency of three times per week, significant improvement was noted with near-complete clearance of most lesions without any adverse effects. The frequency of the phototherapy sessions was therefore reduced to twice weekly initially, and then to once weekly. The patient's disease remained well-controlled for 9 months on once-weekly nbUVB sessions, with the only residual areas of involvement being the feet bilaterally. The patient was then started on a nbUVB home phototherapy kit three times per week for the persistent feet lesions. The patient remained on this regimen for another 12 months as maintenance therapy with gradual resolution of the feet lesions while the rest of the body remained in remission.

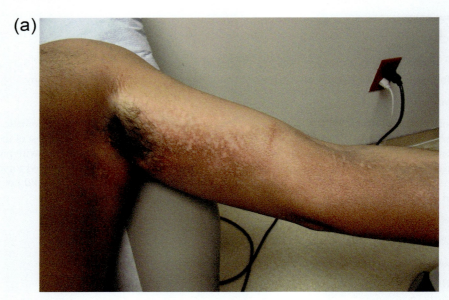

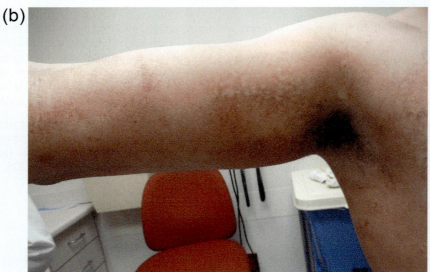

FIGURE 4.4.1 (a and b) Reticulate atrophic erythematous patches with hyper/hypopigmentation and telangiectasias on the bilateral axillae.

Discussion

- Poikilodermatous mycosis fungoides (pMF), also known as poikiloderma atrophicans vascularis, is a rare subtype of MF, comprising approximately 11% of all cases.[1] pMF often presents at a younger age compared to classic MF and has a slight male predominance (male:female ratio of 1.6:1).[1] It is characterized by the clinical triad of telangiectasia, atrophy, and mottled hyper and hypopigmentation, usually arising on the flexural surfaces of the body and trunk.[1]

- Considerable delay in establishing diagnosis is common, with a study reporting a median duration of 10 years before pMF was confirmed.[1] Despite the delay, 92% of patients remained early stage (IIA or less) at the time of diagnosis.[1] The majority were stage I specifically (39% stage IA disease, 47% stage IB disease) and none had stage IV disease.[1]

- The histologic features usually resemble patch/plaque-stage MF. However, the T-cell immuno-phenotype often differs between the two variants.[1] While classic MF is typically CD4+/CD8−, pMF is more commonly CD8+/CD4−, similar to the hypopigmented variant (hMF), both of which are associated with a benign clinical course.[1] Interestingly, both hMF and pMF are also associated with an earlier age of onset (mean 20.6 and 44 years, respectively) compared to classic MF (mean 52–60 years).[1,2]

- First-line treatment for pMF is phototherapy. Various modalities have been utilized to date, including PUVA, ultraviolet B, and nbUVB.[1] In a retrospective study of 49 patients conducted by Abbott et al., 89% of patients (24/27) treated with phototherapy responded to treatment. Of the 18 patients who received PUVA, 15 patients responded to treatment (83%).[1] Additionally, all patients who received UVB (n = 5) and nbUVB (n = 4) responded to treatment.[1] The degree of response was not noted in the study. It is also worth noting that none of the four patients treated with topical corticosteroids responded to treatment, and only 1/4 patients treated with other topical regimens showed a response (including mechlorethamine 0.01%, carmustine 0.04%, and 5-fluorouracil).[1]

- pMF is associated with an excellent overall prognosis.[1,2] In the study by Abbott et al., 96% of the patients remained at the same stage as diagnosis after a mean follow-up period of 11 years and 10 months.[1] Only 2/47 patients progressed, and no patients died of their disease.[1]

Teaching Pearls

- pMF is a rare variant of MF with an overall favorable prognosis
- In comparison to classic MF, pMF appears to be associated with a younger age of onset and is more commonly CD8+/CD4-
- While pMF is often unresponsive to topical regimens, phototherapy can be used effectively in this variant with data from a small study suggesting that nbUVB may have an even better response that PUVA. Additionally, nbUVB has a superior long-term safety profile than PUVA and may therefore be the better choice for first-line therapy in pMF.

References

1. Abbott RA, Sahni D, Robson A, et al. Poikilodermatous mycosis fungoides: a study of its clinicopathological, immunophenotypic, and prognostic features. *J Am Acad Dermatol*. 2011;65(2):313–319.
2. Phan K, Ramachandran V, Fassihi H, et al. Comparison of narrowband UV-B with psoralen-UV-A phototherapy for patients with early-stage mycosis fungoides: a systematic review and meta-analysis. *JAMA Dermatol*. 2019;155(3):335–341.

Case 4.5

Authors: Shreya Patel, MD, Bilal Fawaz, MD, and Michael A. Dyer, MD.

Reason for Presentation: Radiation therapy for effective treatment of palmoplantar MF.

Chief Complaint: Rash on the hands and feet.

History of Present Illness: A middle-aged patient presented with a 4-month history of a painful, itchy rash, which began on the feet and later spread to the hands. The patient stated he regularly used harsh chemicals while cleaning at work, and believed the rash started after coming in contact with bleach. Around 1 month prior to presentation, the rash also spread to involve the elbows and shins. Multiple topical therapies had been tried previously and failed, including clobetasol propionate 0.05% cream, ketoconazole 2% cream, ammonium lactate 12% cream, and clotrimazole cream.

The patient was originally diagnosed with palmoplantar psoriasis with possible superimposed contact dermatitis and had been prescribed oral acitretin, halobetasol 0.05% ointment, and urea 40% cream. Due to insurance issues, however, the patient only used the topical therapies leading to only mild improvement. At the 1-month follow-up visit, the patient's buttocks, bilateral hips, and thighs were noted to be involved with an itchy rash, and a skin biopsy was performed.

Review of Systems: No pertinent positives.

Medical/Surgical History: None.

Medications: Halobetasol 0.05% ointment twice daily; urea 40% cream once nightly.

Family History: No family history of skin cancer or psoriasis.

Social History: Denied smoking, alcohol or illicit drug use; worked as a cleaner.

Physical Examination: Skin type IV; Bilateral palms: Mild-to-moderate hyperkeratosis and desquamation, with well-defined, pink-tan, thin plaques with multiple fissures (Figure 4.5.1a); Bilateral soles: Thick, well-demarcated, deeply fissured hyperkeratotic plaques (Figure 4.5.1b); Trunk and extremities: Several irregular dull pink scaly papules coalescing into larger plaques, body surface area (BSA) ~8%; No palpable lymphadenopathy.

Pathology: Incisional biopsy from a plaque on the right hip (Figure 4.5.2): (A) Focal band-like atypical lymphocytic infiltrate with involvement of both eccrine duct (H&E, 40×) and (B) eccrine coil (H&E, 200×). Lesional cells are positive for (C) CD3 (200×) and (d) CD4 (200×).

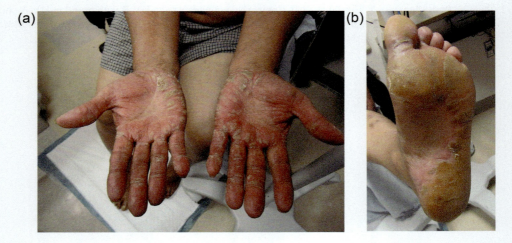

(a)   (b)

FIGURE 4.5.1   (a) Indurated erythematous plaques with focal areas of hyperkeratosis on the bilateral palms, and (b) well-demarcated, yellow, fissured plaques on the left plantar surface with background erythema.

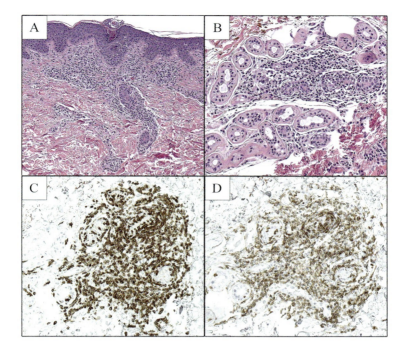

FIGURE 4.5.2 Incisional biopsy from a plaque on the right hip: (A) H&E, 40×; (B) H&E, 200×; (C) positive immunostaining for CD3 (200×); and (d) positive immunostaining for CD4 (200×).

Final Diagnosis: Mycosis fungoides palmaris et plantaris, with evidence of syringotropism, stage IA (T1N0M0B0 at diagnosis).

Management and Disease Course: The patient's systemic evaluation (CBC with differential, CMP, and LDH) was unremarkable, but the tumor burden increased to involve a BSA of 15% at a subsequent follow-up visit (T2bN0M0B0; stage IB). Given the progression, oral bexarotene (150 mg daily initially, slowly uptitrated to 300 mg daily), fenofibrate 160 mg daily, and topical triamcinolone 0.1% ointment were initiated. The patient responded well to the regimen with resolution of the body rash and improvement in the palmoplantar rash after 3 months of therapy. However, the development of marked hypertriglyceridemia (>500 mg/dL) on high-dose bexarotene necessitated a significant dose reduction to 150 mg daily, as well as the addition of omega-3 fatty acids (2 g daily) to fenofibrate.

The change in dosing led to a flare of the palmoplantar disease which once again became fissured and painful. Given the tolerance issues with the higher-dose bexarotene, the cutaneous oncology tumor board panel recommended focal low-dose radiation therapy to the patient's hands and feet. This was given as 8 Gy in two fractions to each of four areas: Right hand, left hand, right foot, and left foot. The four sites were treated sequentially to avoid synchronous radiation dermatitis of the bilateral hands and feet together and difficulty with day-to-day activities. Two to three months following radiation treatment, the symptoms improved considerably. Some disease recurrence in the right foot necessitated retreatment with 24 Gy in 12 fractions. Other than short-lived, moderate radiation dermatitis of 2 months, the patient had a CR of the palmoplantar disease to radiation therapy after which he was lost to follow-up.

Discussion

- Palmoplantar involvement occurs in approximately 12% of patients with MF. However, mycosis fungoides palmaris et plantaris (MFPP), defined by MF limited to or initially presenting on the palms and/or soles, affects only about 0.6% of all MF patients. Although it tends to have an indolent course, it can be difficult to treat.[1]

- The morphologic presentation varies considerably ranging from erythematous, scaly, fissured plaques to vesiculopustular and hyperkeratotic presentations.[2,3] This MF variant is commonly misdiagnosed given its striking resemblance to eczematous and psoriasiform rashes.[2,3] Establishing the diagnosis may be delayed due to treatment overlap as MFPP may respond to therapies usually prescribed for psoriasis, atopic dermatitis, and contact dermatitis.[4]
- Various treatments have been reported to be effective in MFPP and other types of MF with palmoplantar involvement, largely based on case reports or series. Partial remissions have been found using topical or systemic glucocorticoids, phototherapy (UVA and nbUVB), PUVA, topical nitrogen mustard, systemic methotrexate, excimer laser, and surgical excision.[3–5]
- Localized radiotherapy (RT) is an excellent treatment option for this often-refractory entity.[3–6] MF is considered to be a radiosensitive neoplasm and unilesional MF can be treated definitively with focal radiation 20–30 Gy in 1.8 Gy or 2 Gy daily fractions.[6,7] RT is an attractive modality in MFPP given the limited success achieved with other therapies.[3–6] Although MFPP is responsive to relatively low doses of radiation, the need for retreatment is common.[3,5–7]
- In terms of radiation field size and dose, low-dose radiation therapy to a focal area, for example, 8 Gy in two fractions of 4 Gy each, is reasonably effective, with CR rates over 90%.[7] Low-dose RT can be repeated, or if resistant or recurrent disease presents in a particular area, higher doses of 20–30 Gy can be given. The higher doses are associated with better long-term local control but needs to be balanced with the risks of long-term side effects, specifically, skin atrophy, telangiectasia, paresthesia, and muscle cramping when hands and feet are treated.[5–7]

Teaching Pearls

- MFPP is a rare variant of MF that differs from classic MF in its clinical presentation and prognosis; palmoplantar involvement of MF without actually meeting criteria for MFPP is more common.
- Diagnosing MFPP is challenging as it often mimics eczematous or psoriasiform processes. It also tends to be refractory to many treatment modalities.
- MFPP currently lacks evidenced-based treatment guidelines, but radiotherapy is an excellent local treatment option. Low doses can be used effectively and radiation can be repeated if needed.

References

1. Resnik K, Kantor G, Lessin S, et al. Mycosis fungoides palmaris et plantaris. *Arch Dermatol.* 1995;131:1052–1056.
2. Kim J, Foster R, Lam M, et al. Mycosis fungoides: an important differential diagnosis for acquired palmoplantar keratoderma. *Aust J Dermatol.* 2015;56:49–51.
3. Nakai N, Hagura A, Yamazato S, et al. Mycosis fungoides palmaris et plantaris successfully treated with radiotherapy: case report and mini-review of the published work. *J Dermatol.* 2014;41:63–67.
4. Spieth K, Grundmann-Kollmann M, Runne U, et al. Mycosis-fungoides-type cutaneous T cell lymphoma of the hands and soles: a variant causing delay in diagnosis and adequate treatment of patients with palmoplantar eczema. *Dermatology.* 2002;205:239–244.
5. Wang CM, Duvic M, Dabaja BS. Acral erosive mycosis fungoides: successful treatment with localised radiotherapy. *BMJ Case Rep.* 2013; 2013: bcr2012007120 .
6. Hoppe RT. Mycosis fungoides: radiation therapy. *Dermatol Ther.* 2003;16:347–354.
7. Specht L, Dabaja B, Illidge T, et al. Modern radiation therapy for primary cutaneous lymphomas: field and dose guidelines from the International Lymphoma Radiation Oncology Group. *Int J Radiat Oncol Biol Phys.* 2015;92:32–39.

Case 4.6

Authors: Marguerite Sullivan, MD, Sara Al Janahi MD, MSc, Iman Fatima Khan, MS, MPH, Ali Al-Haseni, MD, and Adam Lerner, MD.

Reason for Presentation: Treatment of severe LyP and primary C-ALCL with brentuximab vedotin.

Chief Complaint: New and sudden-onset widespread rash.

History of Present Illness: A middle-aged patient presented with a 2-month history of widespread rash affecting the entire body that started as a red bump on the back. Some lesions healed by themselves, but new ones continued to develop simultaneously. Lesions were slightly itchy and burning in sensation, with larger ones being tender to touch.

Review of Systems: Positive for fatigue. Denied fevers, night sweat, chills, and weight loss.

Medical/Surgical History: Nil relevant.

Medications: Nil relevant.

Social: Nil relevant.

Family History: Nil relevant.

Physical Examination: Skin type I; Face/neck: Mostly on mid-face were smooth firm erythematous papules and small nodules, some with collarettes of scale at the upper lip and lateral face; Trunk and extremities: Scattered numerous erythematous firm (some tender) papules, plaques, and nodules, many with desquamating collarettes of scale and hemorrhagic crust (Figure 4.6.1). Lesions at all stages of evolution throughout body, sparing only the genitalia, palms, and soles. The largest nodule on the upper abdomen was 3 × 2 cm in diameter; lymph nodes: Four <1 cm mobile non-tender nodes in bilateral inguinal area. No cervical/axillary nodes.

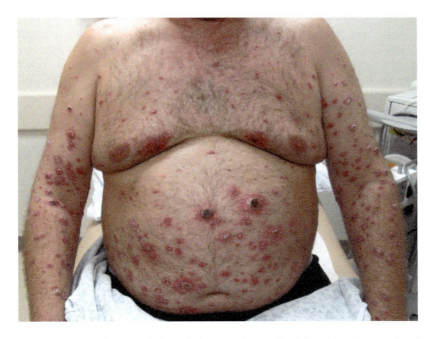

FIGURE 4.6.1 Innumerable erythematous indurated plaques and crusted nodules with collarettes of scale on the chest, abdomen, and upper extremities.

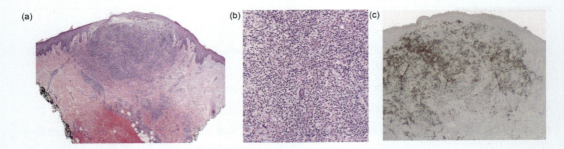

FIGURE 4.6.2   Incisional biopsy from a papule on the right arm: (a) H&E, 10×; (b) H&E, 200×; and (c) positive CD30 immunoperoxidase stain.

Pathology: Incisional biopsy from a papule on the right arm revealed a wedge-shaped superficial and deep perivascular and interstitial lymphohistiocytic infiltrate with scattered neutrophils and extravasated erythrocytes; immunostaining was positive for CD30 (Figure 4.6.2).

Final Diagnosis: LyP.

Management and Disease Course: The patient was started on methotrexate 10 mg weekly with folic acid 1 mg daily. The following month this dose was increased to 15 mg per week with associated improvement in the lesions. Despite the fact that most lesions began to resolve, one lesion on the back enlarged rapidly and developed an ulcerated tumor (Figure 4.6.3).

An incisional biopsy from this lesion demonstrated a dense sheet-like infiltrate of large atypical cells (Figure 4.6.4A). Tumor cells were CD30-positive (Figure 4.6.4B) and ALK-negative, which confirmed the diagnosis of ALK-negative anaplastic large T-cell lymphoma (ALK-negative ALCL).

Staging PET-CT of the whole body showed no evidence of systemic disease and confirmed the diagnosis of PC-ALCL. A further increase in the dose of the methotrexate to 20 mg weekly made little difference and the patient continued to develop more enlarging, ulcerating nodules. Biopsy of the new nodules confirmed more lesions of PC-ALCL, making his presentation that of multifocal PC-ALCL.

Subsequently, the patient's therapy was switched to brentuximab vedotin 1.8 mg/kg every 3 weeks. The large tumor on the back shrank in size after the first week of therapy; after four cycles of brentuximab, it completely resolved. The widespread lesions of LyP that had been shrinking in size on methotrexate previously now fully resolved on brentuximab. Therapy was then stopped. Two months after stopping therapy, the LyP lesions (but not the PC-ALCL) recurred and methotrexate was re-initiated at 15 mg weekly. This dose of methotrexate kept the LyP under excellent long-term control for over 5 years with no recurrence of the PC-ALCL.

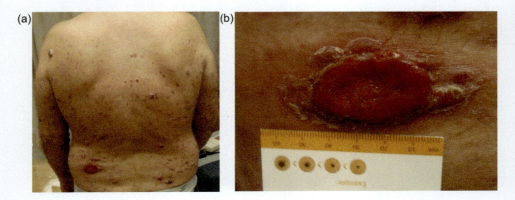

FIGURE 4.6.3   (a and b) Friable, macerated, erythematous, ulcerated tumor with irregular borders and a collarette of scale on the left lower back; note the background papulonodules are involuting.

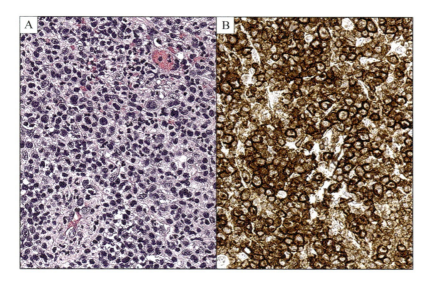

FIGURE 4.6.4 Incisional biopsy of the left lower back nodule: (A) H&E, 400× and (B) positive immunoperoxidase staining for CD30, 400×.

Discussion

- Primary cutaneous CD30+ T-cell lymphoproliferative disorders are the second most common type of CTCL. These encompass a spectrum of related diseases that includes LyP, PC-ALCL, and borderline lesions.[1]

- LyP presents as chronic, recurrent crops of red to violaceous papules and nodules <2 cm that regress spontaneously over 1–3 months leaving behind hypopigmented scars or hyperpigmented macules. Although LyP has an excellent prognosis, these patients are at increased risk for developing a second lymphoid malignancy in ~20% cases. Most commonly, the second malignancy is MF, PC-ALCL, or Hodgkin's lymphoma.[1]

- PC-ALCL presents as rapidly growing red to violaceous solitary nodules or, more rarely, multifocal nodules as in our case. Lesions of PC-ALCL are typically large tumors >2 cm which are known to show regression in many cases, but usually do not resolve fully like LyP.[1] Before making a diagnosis of PC-ALCL, it is critical to rule out an underlying diagnosis of systemic ALCL with cutaneous spread, which has a worse prognosis and different management approach. The ALK-1 staining is helpful though not absolutely reliable in doing this. ALK-1 is a fusion protein formed by a t(2;5) chromosomal translocation that is often present in systemic ALCL. ALK-1 staining is therefore often positive in systemic ALCL but negative in PC-ALCL.[2] However, 40%–50% of systemic ALCL has been demonstrated to be ALK-1 negative, and there are reports of PC-ALCL being ALK-1 positive. Hence, it is essential to follow-up pathological stains with CT or PET-CT scans to rule out systemic disease. Of note, ~10%–15% cases of PC-ALCL may progress to extracutaneous spread, most commonly to regional lymph nodes.[2]

- Brentuximab vedotin is an anti-CD30 antibody which is conjugated to monomethyl auristatin E (MMAE). CD30 is a cell membrane protein in the TNF receptor family that is expressed by a variety of lymphoid malignancies. Upon binding CD30, the antibody-drug conjugate is internalized into the cell. Here, MMAE, an inhibitor of microtubule polymerization, is subsequently cleaved from the antibody and causes cell cycle arrest and apoptosis.[3]

- A phase II study of brentuximab showed an overall response rate of 73% and CR rate of 35% for CD30+ MF. A 100% response rate was observed in LyP and PC-ALCL. Responses occurred within 3 weeks for LyP and PC-ALCL and 12 weeks for MF.[3]

- In the phase III study comparing physicians' choice of methotrexate or bexarotene versus brentuximab, the objective global response rate lasting at least 4 months was 56.3% with brentuximab versus 12.5% with physicians' choice of bexarotene or methotrexate, with similar rates of serious adverse events.[4] Brentuximab vedotin was FDA-approved in 2017 for use in PC-ALCL and CD30-expressing MF that had been previously treated with at least one systemic therapy. It is administered intravenously at a dose of 1.8 mg/kg every 3 weeks until a maximum of 16 cycles, disease progression, or unacceptable toxicity. Brentuximab should be avoided in patients with severe hepatic impairment.
- Peripheral neuropathy is the most commonly reported adverse effect for brentuximab affecting ~60%–70% of patients.[4,5] It is typically associated with a mild distal sensory neuropathy which presents with numbness and tingling in the fingers and toes. This is caused by the toxic effect of MMAE on axonal microtubules. However, more severe motor neuropathy effects can also occur and have been reported in ~10% of patients in previous trials with brentuximab.[5] The exact etiology for the motor neuropathy is unclear but is associated with an inflammatory demyelinating polyradiculopathy that can resemble Guillain–Barré syndrome or CIDP (chronic inflammatory demyelinating polyradiculopathy). It is essential to refer patients developing motor symptoms on brentuximab therapy to neurology for urgent nerve conduction studies and consideration of immune therapy for treatment. The development of neuropathy may require temporary or permanent withdrawal of therapy, which usually though not always, leads to reversal of symptoms.[5] Fatigue, nausea, rash, and neutropenia were other commonly reported adverse effects of brentuximab vedotin.

Teaching Pearls

- Brentuximab vedotin is an anti-CD30 antibody-drug conjugate that provides a relatively safe, effective alternative therapy for patients with severe LyP or PC-ALCL who have failed prior systemic therapy. It is also a treatment option for CD30-expressing MF.
- It is important to check for peripheral neuropathy in patients on brentuximab therapy and alter the drug regimen accordingly if this toxicity develops.

References

1. Kartan S, Johnson W, Sokol K, et al. The spectrum of CD30 T cell lymphoproliferative disorders in the skin. *Chin Clin Oncol*. 2019;8(1):3.
2. Stoll JR, Willner J, Oh Y, et al. Primary cutaneous T-cell lymphomas other than Mycosis Fungoides and Sezary Syndrome - Part I: clinical and histologic features and diagnosis. *J Am Acad Dermatol*. 2021 Nov;85(5):1073–1090.
3. Duvic M, Tetzlaff MT, Gangar P, et al. Results of a Phase II Trial of Brentuximab Vedotin for CD30+ Cutaneous T-Cell Lymphoma and Lymphomatoid Papulosis. *J Clin Oncol*. 2015;33:3759.
4. Prince HM, Kim YH, Horwitz SM, et al. Brentuximab vedotin or physician's choice in CD30-positive cutaneous T-cell lymphoma (ALCANZA): an international, open-label, randomised, phase 3, multicentre trial. *Lancet*. 2017;390(10094):555–566.
5. Fargeot G, Dupel-Pottier C, Stephant M, et al. Brentuximab vedotin treatment associated with acute and chronic inflammatory demyelinating polyradiculoneuropathies. *J Neurol Neurosurg Psychiat*. 2020;91(7):786–788.

Case 4.7

Authors: Yasin Damji, MD, Bilal Fawaz, MD, and Adam Lerner, MD.

Reason for Presentation: Management of advanced primary cutaneous follicle center B-cell lymphoma (PCFCL).

Chief Complaint: Numerous scalp lesions.

History of Present Illness: A young healthy patient was noted to have two asymptomatic bumps on his scalp on a routine physical examination which were of 2-year duration. The patient was referred to dermatology, but was lost to follow-up and presented to our department 1 year later with five additional scalp lesions.

Review of Systems: No pertinent positives.

Medical/Surgical History: None.

Medications: None.

Family History: Nil relevant.

Social History: Non-smoker.

Physical Examination: Skin type IV; Right parietal scalp: 1.0×1.5 cm red-brown firm dermal nodule; Left parietal scalp: Four red-brown, firm, dermal nodules, varying in size from 1 to 3 cm (Figure 4.7.1); Similar nodules were noted on the upper back; Right axilla: One small palpable mobile lymph node on the right posterior axillary vault.

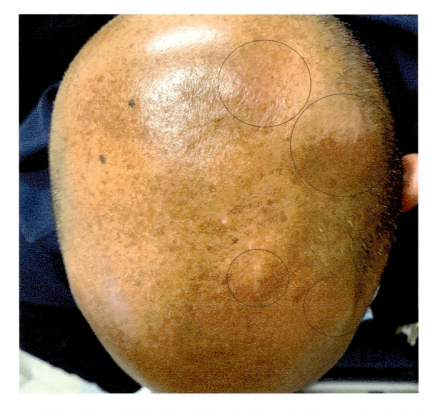

FIGURE 4.7.1 Multiple, red-brown, ill-defined, firm, indurated nodules on the left vertex and parietal scalp.

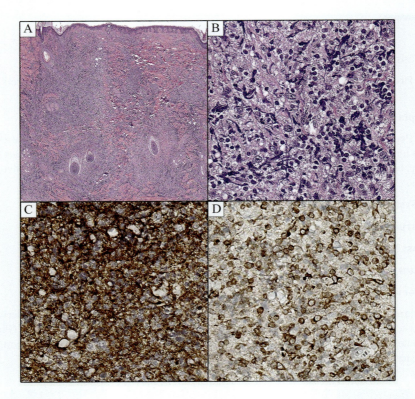

FIGURE 4.7.2 Incisional biopsy of the right lateral back nodule: (A) H&E, 20×; (B) H&E, 400×; (C) positive immunostaining for CD10 (400×); and (D) positive immunostaining for BCL6 (400×).

Pathology: Incisional biopsy of the right lateral back nodule (Figure 4.7.2): (A) A dense, superficial and deep, nodular, periappendageal, and interstitial lymphocytic infiltrate (H&E, 20×); (B) higher power demonstrating B-cells with a centrocyte, centroblast, and immunoblast morphology (H&E, 400×). In addition to CD20, lesional cells are positive with immunoperoxidase staining for (C) CD10 (400×) and (D) BCL6 (400×).

Investigations

- CBC, CMP, and LDH all within normal limits.
- **HIV:** Negative.
- **HTLV-1:** Negative.
- Flow cytometric analysis of peripheral blood showed only a minor polytypic B-cell population (accounting for 10% of all nucleated cells), suggesting no peripheral blood involvement.
- CT chest, abdomen, and pelvis with contrast: No evidence of systemic disease.
- Bone marrow biopsy: No evidence of marrow involvement.

Final Diagnosis: PCFCL, T2aN0M0.

Management and Disease Course

After biopsy confirmation of the patient's PCFCL, the case was discussed at the cutaneous oncology tumor board and local radiation was recommended. However, the patient was again lost to follow-up and later presented again with an additional biopsy-confirmed lesion of PCFCL on his back. Given the disease progression to more extensive skin involvement, systemic therapy with rituximab was started (375 mg/m^2 IV weekly × 4 weeks initially, followed by every 2 months for maintenance therapy × 1 year). The patient responded to rituximab with resolution of his disease. Two years later, a new scalp lesion developed with skin biopsy confirming PCFCL recurrence. He was restarted on another 1-year course of rituximab with CR.

Discussion

- PCFCL classically presents as firm, erythematous, painless plaques and tumors on the head or trunk. Histology demonstrates large follicle center cells with centrocytes and centroblasts arranged in follicular, follicular and diffuse, or diffuse patterns. Cells express B-lymphocyte markers CD19, CD20, and CD79a and the germinal cell marker Bcl-6; neoplastic cells also specifically express CD10 in this form of cutaneous lymphoma.[1]
- PCFCL is usually indolent and rarely metastasizes, giving it a good prognosis overall. Due to this indolent nature, localized radiotherapy (30 Gy) is often the first-line treatment of limited cutaneous disease.[2] In one of the largest studies to date, indolent CBCLs, including PCFCL and PCMZL, were associated with a 98% local control rate after monotherapy with radiation.[2]
- In cases with more extensive disease, systemic therapy is often recommended, most commonly with rituximab.[1] Rituximab is a monoclonal antibody that binds to the CD20 antigen on B-lymphocytes, resulting in multiple mechanisms of induced cell death including NK-cell-mediated antibody-dependent cellular cytotoxicity (ADCC). In a recent retrospective review of 18 patients with CBCL, including 11 patients with PCFCL, 10/11 patients (90.9%) demonstrated an initial CR to rituximab.[3] However, recurrences were common (81.8%), necessitating radiotherapy or repeat rituximab therapy. No long-term follow-up was available. Intralesional administration of rituximab (median dose of 150 mg per lesion) has also resulted in complete resolution of lesions.[1,2]
- Despite reports of cutaneous relapse, rituximab therapy was well-tolerated and no severe adverse effects were reported in PCFCL patients after a median follow-up time of 52 months.[3] Rituximab is considered to be a safe and efficacious treatment option for patients who are not candidates for radiotherapy or for patients with extensive cutaneous involvement.[3]

Teaching Pearls

- PCFCL is an indolent CBCL that rarely metastasizes and has an overall good prognosis.
- Radiotherapy may be used for localized disease.
- Rituximab is a safe and effective option when patients have extensive disease. Though disease recurrence is common, repeat treatment can be given.

References

1. Vermeer MH, Willemze R. Recent advances in primary cutaneous B-cell lymphomas. *Curr Opin Oncol.* 2014;26(2):230–236.
2. Hamilton SN, Wai ES, Tan K, et al. Treatment and outcomes in patients with primary cutaneous B-cell lymphoma: the BC cancer agency experience. *Int J Radiat Oncol Biol Phys.* 2013;87:719–725.
3. Brandenburg A, Humme D, Terhorst D, et al. Long-term outcome of intravenous therapy with rituximab in patients with primary cutaneous B-cell lymphomas. *Br J Dermatol.* 2013;169(5):1126–1132.

Case 4.8

Authors: Emily Coleman, MD, Bilal Fawaz, MD, and Adam Lerner, MD.

Reason for Presentation: Successful treatment of PC-DLBCL, leg-type with reduced dose R-CHOP in an elderly patient.

Chief Complaint: Rash on right leg.

History of Present Illness: An elderly woman presented to dermatology for a several month history of a lesion on the right shin. She did not respond to terbinafine hydrochloride cream prescribed by an outside provider. Over the subsequent 2 months, her lesion began to enlarge and progress in this area but was otherwise asymptomatic.

Review of Systems: No pertinent positives.

Medical/Surgical History: Prior breast cancer s/p surgery, adjuvant chemotherapy, and hormonal therapy (cyclophosphamide, adriamycin, 5-fluorouracil, exemestane, tamoxifen).

Medications: Omeprazole 40 mg as needed; metoprolol succinate 100 mg daily; enalapril 20 mg; amlodipine-atorvastatin 5–20 mg once daily; lorazepam 0.5 mg as needed; duloxetine 60 mg daily; temazepam 7.5 mg as needed.

Family History: Nil relevant.

Social History: Former smoker (10 pack-year history); denied alcohol or illicit drug use;

Physical Examination: Skin type II; Right medial lower leg: Numerous, clustered indurated red-brown arcuate-polycyclic plaques (Figure 4.8.1); Scattered dome-shaped nodules on the right lower extremity; No palpable lymphadenopathy.

Pathology: Biopsy of the right lower leg plaque (Figure 4.8.2): (a) Diffuse dermal and subcutaneous infiltrate; (b) sheet-like proliferation of atypical, large, round, hyperchromatic lymphocytes with numerous mitoses; immunoperoxidase staining reveals the tumor cells to be positive for (c) CD20 and (d) MUM-1.

Investigations

- **White blood cells:** 11.4 K/µL (reference range: 4.0–11.0 K/µL); absolute lymphocytes 4.0 K/µL (reference range: 1.1–3.5 K/µL).
- **PET/CT:** 0.6 cm left submandibular lymph node with an SUV max of 5.6 cm; uptake within the bilateral glenohumeral joint spaces, consistent with severe arthritis; prominent joint effusion seen in the right shoulder; focal uptake in the right posterior medial calf with associated nodular skin thickening with an SUV of 9.7.
- **Localization CT scan:** Hepatomegaly with cephalocaudal extent of 20 cm; the spleen is absent.

Final Diagnosis: Stage IE primary cutaneous diffuse large B-cell lymphoma, leg-type (PC-DLBCL).

Management and Disease Course: After biopsy confirmation of PC-DLBCL, PET/CT showed what were likely reactive lymphadenopathy. The patient was hesitant about undergoing chemotherapy due to her advanced age and her past morbid experience with chemotherapy for breast cancer. Therefore, the decision was made to start the patient on dose-reduced R-CHOP, in which the CHOP doses are halved (rituximab 375 mg/m^2; cyclophosphamide 400 mg/m^2; doxorubicin 25 mg/m^2; vincristine 1 mg; and prednisone 40 mg/m^2 on days 1–5). She successfully completed six cycles of the regimen at 3-week intervals.

The patient subsequently received six fractions of consolidative radiation therapy with a total dose of 28.50 Gy. Follow-up PET/CT showed no abnormal FDG uptake. Unfortunately, the patient developed congestive heart failure following her chemotherapy course despite a lifetime cumulative anthracycline dose of 300 mg/m^2. She remains without recurrence of her PC-DLBCL 5 years after diagnosis.

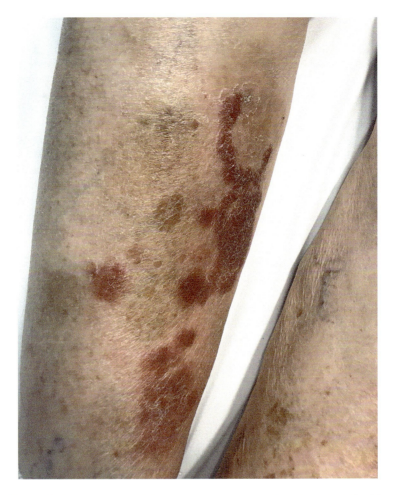

FIGURE 4.8.1 Clustered, well-demarcated, red-brown, arcuate-polycylic, indurated plaques on the right medial lower leg.

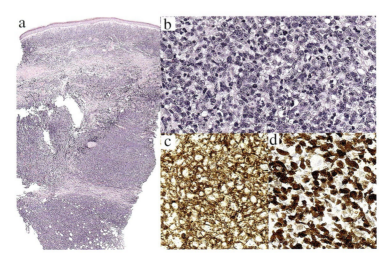

FIGURE 4.8.2 Biopsy of the right lower leg plaque: (a) H&E, 10×; (b) H&E, 400×; (c) immunoperoxidase staining for CD20 (400×); and (d) immunoperoxidase staining for MUM-1 (400×).

Discussion

- Primary cutaneous diffuse large B-cell lymphoma, leg-type (PC-DLBCL) is a type of cutaneous B-cell lymphoma characterized by rapidly progressive cutaneous tumors with a high rate of systemic involvement.[1] It most commonly presents on the lower legs, but up to 20% of cases involve other anatomical sites, such as the upper extremities and trunk.[1] The median age at presentation is 70–82 years, with a female predominance. Extracutaneous spread of PC-DLBCL is typical, and prognosis is usually poor with a 5-year overall survival of <60%.[1]

- Histologically, PC-DLBCL is characterized by diffuse sheets of immunoblasts and centroblasts with deep extension into the dermis and subcutis, typically sparing the epidermis.[1] It demonstrates high rates of bcl-2, MUM-1, and FOX-P1 positivity, and co-expression of c-myc portends a worse prognosis than PC-DLBCL expressing bcl-2 alone.[1]

- Given the poor outcomes in PC-DLBCL, first-line therapy is usually systemic chemotherapy with or without radiation.[1,2] Specifically, rituximab, cyclophosphamide, hydroxydaunorubicin (doxorubicin or adriamycin), oncovin (vincristine), and prednisone (i.e., R-CHOP) is most commonly recommended.[1,2]

- R-CHOP often has significant adverse effects (AEs) in elderly patients with comorbidities.[1] Interestingly, one study found that decreasing the dose of CHOP by half (so-called R-miniCHOP) in patients over 80 years old led to acceptable efficacy with more tolerable side effects.[4] The reported 2-year overall survival was 59%, with a median overall survival of 29 months.[4] This study was pivotal to our decision planning in this case, given the patient's age and concern about the potential for adverse effects of full-dose chemotherapy. R-miniCHOP may, therefore, be a suitable alternative to R-CHOP in elderly patients with comorbidities, although the decision to reduce chemotherapy doses in this fashion is best made on a case-by-case basis.[4]

Teaching Pearls

- PC-DLBCL is an aggressive CBCL with high propensity for extracutaneous metastasis. It primarily affects elderly patients who often have comorbidities that limit the tolerability of R-CHOP, the standard of care for this lymphoma.

- Dose-reduced R-CHOP, or R-miniCHOP, should be considered in DLBCL patients over 80 years of age, given its superior tolerability when compared to R-CHOP.[3]

References

1. Wilcox RA. Cutaneous B-cell lymphomas: 2019 update on diagnosis, risk stratification, and management. *Am J Hematol.* 2018;93(11):1427–1430.
2. Jia J, Li W, Zheng Y. Primary cutaneous diffuse large B cell lymphomaother successfully treated by the combination of R-CHOP chemotherapy and surgery A case report and review of literature. *Medicine (Baltimore).* 2017 Feb;96(8):e6161.
3. Peyrade F, Jardin F, Thieblemont C, et al. Attenuated immunochemotherapy regimen (R-miniCHOP) in elderly patients older than 80 years with diffuse large B-cell lymphoma: a multicentre, single-arm, phase 2 trial. *Lancet Oncol.* 2011;12(5):460–468.

5

Kaposi's Sarcoma

Bilal Fawaz and Debjani Sahni

CONTENTS

Introduction

Kaposi's sarcoma (KS) is a rare angioproliferative neoplasm that presents in a variety of clinical settings.[1-3] A common feature to all variants is the association with human herpesvirus-8 (HHV-8), which is thought to play an essential role in its pathogenesis.[1] The four principal clinical variants include classic KS, African-endemic KS, KS due to iatrogenic immunosuppression, and acquired immunodeficiency syndrome (AIDS)-associated epidemic KS.[2,3] More recently, a fifth variant, termed non-epidemic KS, has been increasingly reported in young, otherwise healthy men who have sex with men (MSM). Non-epidemic KS patients lack the other risk factors typically associated with KS and appear to have a favorable prognosis overall.[4]

In 1872, Moritz Kaposi first described KS in five men as "idiopathic multiple pigmented sarcomas of the skin", now considered the classic variant.[5] Classic KS commonly presents on the lower extremities of elderly men of Mediterranean, Eastern European, or Ashkenazi Jewish descent.[2-5] The majority of cases present after the age of 50 years, with one study reporting a median age of 67 years in men and 64 years in females.[6] Prognosis is generally thought to be favorable, with patients surviving an average of 10–15 years before dying of unrelated causes.[2]

African-endemic KS similarly has a clear male predominance, with an estimated incidence of ~1%–10% among black Africans.[2,7] It is further subdivided into four categories: Nodular, florid, infiltrative, and lymphadenopathic.[2] The lymphadenopathic variant is notable in that it usually develops in the pediatric population and primarily affects lymph nodes.[8] It also differs from most KS variants because of its fulminant course, with most patients succumbing to their disease within 2–3 years.[2,8]

Iatrogenic KS develops due to chronic immunosuppression, most commonly in the setting of organ transplantation and inflammatory disorders.[3] This variant has a slight male predominance with an estimated incidence of 0.5%–5.3% among transplant patients.[9,10] The disease arises after an average of 16–31 months post-transplant.[3,9-11] The most commonly implicated agents are cyclosporine and corticosteroids.[11] If untreated, iatrogenic KS tends to be aggressive with significant visceral involvement. Management of this type of KS has a three-pronged approach involving reduction or withdrawal of immunosuppression and switching to a mammalian target of rapamycin (mTOR) inhibitor or chemotherapy. Iatrogenic KS often poses a management dilemma as reducing immunosuppression may not be feasible and can lead to transplant rejection or end-organ damage, depending on the underlying condition.[9-11]

DOI: 10.1201/9780429026683-5

Epidemic KS has long been one of the most frequently diagnosed AIDS-defining illnesses, and it remains the most common AIDS-associated neoplasm in the United States today.[2,3] Approximately 95% of cases present in MSM at a mean age of 37 years and an age range of 18–65 years.[2] Advanced immune impairment is often required for its development as CD4+ counts <200 cells/µL are often noted on presentation.[12] A CD4+:CD8+ ratio <0.5 was recently proposed to be the best marker for KS risk, independent of CD4+ count.[12]

Significant clinical and histologic overlap exists between all variants. The disease often begins with pink-violaceous-brown macules, patches, and plaques, which may progress to form larger nodules and tumors.[2,3] Mucosal involvement is frequently present, particularly in the oral cavity.[2] Histologic findings are common to all variants but vary according to stage.[2] Patch/plaque-stage KS presents with a superficial/deep dermal proliferation of angulated vessels and spindled endothelial cells lacking significant atypia or mitoses. A sparse lymphoplasmacytic infiltrate is typically present.[2] In nodular KS, spindled endothelial cells replace dermal collagen and form slit-like vascular spaces with erythrocyte extravasation.[2] Immunohistochemical expression of latency-associated nuclear antigen (LANA-1) of HHV-8 confirms the diagnosis, as it is highly specific and sensitive for KS.[3]

Treatment varies depending on the clinical variant, the degree of involvement, and the patient's overall health status.[3] In immunocompetent, asymptomatic patients with limited disease, observation is reasonable.[3] Withdrawal or reduction of immunosuppression is generally pursued for iatrogenic KS, and antiretroviral therapy is essential for AIDS-associated KS.[10–12] Patients with localized disease may be treated with surgical excision, radiation therapy, photodynamic therapy, cryotherapy, topical alitretinoin or imiquimod, and intralesional chemotherapy.[3] Systemic therapy should be considered in severe or progressive disease, most notably with liposomal anthracyclines, paclitaxel, and, more recently, pomalidomide.[13,14]

References

1. Schulz TF, Cesarman E. Kaposi sarcoma-associated herpesvirus: mechanisms of oncogenesis. *Curr Opin Virol*. 2015;14:116–128.
2. Tappero JW, Conant MA, Wolfe SF, et al. Kaposi's sarcoma. Epidemiology, pathogenesis, histology, clinical spectrum, staging criteria and therapy. *J Am Acad Dermatol*. 1993;28:371–395.
3. Antman K, Chang Y. Kaposi's sarcoma. *N Engl J Med*. 2000;342:1027–1038.
4. Vangipuram R, Tyring SK. Epidemiology of Kaposi sarcoma: review and description of the nonepidemic variant. *Int J Dermatol*. 2019;58(5):538–542.
5. Kaposi M. Idiopathic multiple pigmented sarcoma of the skin. *CA Cancer J Clin*. 1982;32:342–347.
6. DiGiovanna JJ, Safai B. Kaposi's sarcoma: retrospective study of 90 cases with particular emphasis on the familial occurrences, ethnic background and prevalence of other diseases. *Am J Med*. 1981;71:779–783.
7. Taylor JF, Templeton AC, Vogel CL, et al. Kaposi's sarcoma in Uganda: a clinico-pathological study. *Int J Cancer*. 1971;8:122–135.
8. Mittermayer-Vassallo K, Banda K, Molyneux EM. Kaposi sarcoma in HIV-seronegative children presenting to the paediatric oncology ward in the Queen Elizabeth Central Hospital, Blantyre, Malawi during 2002–2014. *Trop Doct*. 2016;46(3):138–142.
9. Penn R. Kaposi's sarcoma in immunosuppressed patients. *J Clin Lab Immunol*. 1983;12:1–10.
10. Lesnoni La Parola I, Masini C, Nanni G, et al. Kaposi's sarcoma in renal-transplant recipients: experience at the Catholic University in Rome, 1988–1996. *Dermatology*. 1997;194:229–233.
11. Brambilla L, Tourlaki A, Genovese G. Iatrogenic Kaposi's sarcoma: a retrospective cohort study in an Italian tertiary care centre. *Clin Oncol*. 2017;29(10):e165–e171.
12. Poizot-Martin I, Lions C, Cheret A, et al. Kaposi sarcoma in people living with HIV: incidence and associated factors in a French cohort between 2010 and 2015. *AIDS*. 2020;1534(4):569–577.
13. Northfelt DW, Dezube BJ, Thommes JA, et al. Pegylated-liposomal doxorubicin versus doxorubicin, bleomycin, and vincristine in the treatment of AIDS-related Kaposi's sarcoma: results of a randomized phase III clinical trial. *J Clin Oncol*. 1998;16(7):2445–2451.
14. Polizzotto MN, Uldrick TS, Wyvill KM, et al. Pomalidomide for Symptomatic Kaposi's sarcoma in people with and without HIV infection: a phase I/II study. *J Clin Oncol*. 2016;34(34):4125–4131.

Case 5.1

Authors: Nicole Patzelt, Tatchai Ruangrattanatavorn, Elizabeth T. Rotrosen, and Adam Lerner.

Reason for Presentation: Management approach to iatrogenic KS.

Chief Complaint: Eye swelling and leg lesions.

History of Present Illness: A 34-year-old Ugandan male who presented with a 1-year history of asymptomatic lesions on the legs, arms, and right cheek, associated with bilateral leg swelling. The patient also had accompanying right eye periorbital swelling for 9 months prior to presentation, without visual disturbance. CT of the head revealed an orbital mass that on biopsy was consistent with KS. He was subsequently referred to the cutaneous oncology clinic for further management.

Review of Systems: No pertinent positives.

Medical/Surgical History: End-stage renal disease s/p renal transplant, cardiomyopathy, and superior vena cava syndrome (related to prior central lines).

Medications: Tacrolimus, mycophenolate mofetil, and lisinopril.

Physical Examination: Face: Right periorbital edema; Right cheek: 1 cm violaceous-hyperpigmented plaque; Bilateral upper and lower extremities: Numerous violaceous-hyperpigmented dermal patches and papules, some coalescing into larger plaques (see Figure 5.1.1); No cervical, axillary, or inguinal lymphadenopathy.

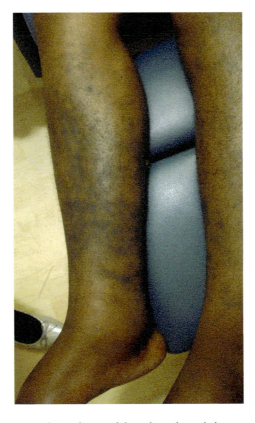

FIGURE 5.1.1   Right leg with numerous hyperpigmented dermal papules and plaques coalescing into larger plaques.

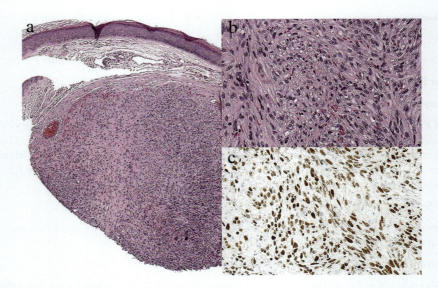

FIGURE 5.1.2   Punch biopsy of a right leg papule: (a) H&E, 100×; (b) H&E, 200×; and (c) positive nuclear staining of tumor cells for human herpesvirus 8.

Pathology: Punch biopsy of a right leg plaque (see Figure 5.1.2): (a) A relatively well-circumscribed dermal mass (H&E, 100×); (b) Interlacing short fascicles of spindle cells with slit-like blood vessels and scattered erythrocytes (H&E, 200×); and (c) Positive nuclear staining of tumor cells for human herpesvirus 8 (200×); consistent with: KS, nodular stage.

Investigations

- HIV testing was negative.
- PET/CT showed multiple hypermetabolic abnormalities consistent with malignant disease including the right orbit; bilateral nodular pleural lesions associated with pleural effusions; supraclavicular, axillary, retroperitoneal, and mesenteric lymphadenopathy; and intra-abdominal ascites concerning for peritoneal disease.

Final Diagnosis: Iatrogenic KS.

Management and Disease Course: The patient was tapered off tacrolimus and started on sirolimus 2 mg daily while continuing mycophenolate 500 mg BID. He had a partial response of his lesions to this regimen at his 2-month follow-up visit. The sirolimus dose was subsequently increased but the patient was unable to tolerate higher doses due to significant gastrointestinal upset. He was switched back to 2 mg daily of sirolimus, but progressive internal KS lesions were noted on CT scan. Hence, PEGylated-liposomal doxorubicin (PLD) was initiated at 20 mg/m² every 3 weeks eventually resulting in a complete response of his disease. After discontinuation of liposomal doxorubicin, he was well-controlled on low-dose sirolimus and mycophenolate mofetil.

Discussion

- KS is classified as iatrogenic/post-transplantation in patients on immunosuppressive therapy. Switching patients from calcineurin inhibitors, such as tacrolimus and cyclosporine, to a mammalian target of rapamycin (mTOR) inhibitor, for example, sirolimus, can improve their KS, as demonstrated in this case.[1]

- Numerous retrospective and prospective studies of post-transplantation KS patients have shown either complete or partial remission of KS lesions in a majority of the patients studied once switched to an mTOR inhibitor.[1–3] Of note, the vast majority of these reports involve cutaneous lesions of KS only, although there are a few reports of improvement in patients with visceral involvement as well.[1–3]

- Stallone et al. demonstrated complete resolution of KS lesions in 15 renal transplant patients after conversion from cyclosporine to sirolimus treatment within 3 months of the treatment change.[1]

- Gutierrez-Dalmau et al. showed that six of their seven renal transplant KS patients had regression of lesions with stable renal function after conversion from calcineurin inhibitors to sirolimus treatment.[2] One patient required hemodialysis due to acute renal failure that was not attributable to conversion to sirolimus, but rather an episode of pneumonia with cardiac failure.[2]

- Whereas calcineurin inhibitors are only immunosuppressive, mTOR inhibitors are both immunosuppressive (accounting for the continued graft acceptance in transplant patients after conversion of therapy) and anti-neoplastic.[3] The mechanism for this has been demonstrated in mouse models where mTOR inhibitors had a direct cytotoxic effect on KS tumor cells by inhibiting angiogenesis.[4] This was achieved by reducing vascular endothelial growth factor secretion and therefore reducing formation of tumor vasculature.[4] mTOR inhibitors may also inhibit tumor cell proliferation by inhibiting IL-2-induced T-cell clonal expansion via inhibition of p70 S6 kinase, which normally stimulates progression through the cell cycle.[5]

- In patients with a partial or lack of response to switching immunosuppressive therapies, adding liposomal doxorubicin can be effective in KS, as demonstrated in this case.[6] Liposomal doxorubicin has the advantage over non-liposomal formulations of this drug by being less toxic (less alopecia and anthracycline-associated cardiotoxicity) as a result of its relatively specific delivery via the liposome to tissues that have "leaky" endothelium, such as tumors. In particular, the relatively low cardiotoxicity of liposomal doxorubicin allows prolonged use of this drug in patients over many years, something that would not be possible with free doxorubicin.

- Calcineurin inhibitors continue to be the mainstay of post-transplant immunosuppressive regimens despite the reports of patients developing KS. This is because calcineurin inhibitors are generally better tolerated than mTOR inhibitors. Common side effects of mTOR inhibitors include hypertriglyceridemia (often requiring dietary and pharmacologic management), anemia, edema, and leg swelling.[1–3] More serious but less common side effects include thrombocytopenia, leukopenia, neutropenia, lymphopenia, amenorrhea, poor wound healing, post-operative lymphoceles, and pneumonitis. Serious side effects are often dose-dependent.[1–3]

Teaching Pearls

- In post-transplant patients who develop KS while on calcineurin inhibitors (such as tacrolimus), conversion of immunosuppressive therapy to mTOR inhibitors (such as sirolimus) can lead to partial or complete resolution of KS lesions.
- Sirolimus acts via an anti-angiogenesis effect on the KS tumor cells.
- If there is an incomplete response of KS lesions after conversion of immune therapy, liposomal doxorubicin is frequently an effective and well-tolerated adjuvant therapy for this disease.

References

1. Stallone G, Schena A, Infante B, et al. Sirolimus for Kaposi's sarcoma in renal-transplant recipients. *N Engl J Med*. 2005;352(13):1317–1323.
2. Gutiérrez-Dalmau A, Sánchez-Fructuoso A, Sanz-Guajardo A, et al. Efficacy of conversion to sirolimus in posttransplantation Kaposi's sarcoma. *Transpl Proc*. 2005;37(9):3836–3838.

3. Mohsin N, Budruddin M, Pakkyarra A, et al. Complete regression of visceral Kaposi's sarcoma after conversion to sirolimus. *Exp Clin Transpl*. 2005;3(2):366–369.
4. Roy D, Sin SH, Lucas A, et al. mTOR inhibitors block Kaposi sarcoma growth by inhibiting essential autocrine growth factors and tumor angiogenesis. *Cancer Res*. 2013;73(7):2235–2246.
5. Thomson AW, Trunquist HR, Raimondi G. Immunoregulatory functions of mTOR inhibition. *Nat Rev Immunol*. 2009;9(5):324–337.
6. Northfelt DW, Dezube BJ, Thommes JA, et al. Pegylated-liposomal doxorubicin versus doxorubicin, bleomycin, and vincristine in the treatment of AIDS-related Kaposi's sarcoma: results of a randomized phase III clinical trial. *J Clin Oncol*. 1998;16(7):2445–2451.

Case 5.2

Authors: Nicole Patzelt, Malathi Chittireddy, Hanna Mumber, and Adam Lerner.

Reason for Presentation: Approach to treating epidemic KS.

Chief Complaint: Bumps on the leg.

History of Present Illness: A young man with a recent diagnosis of hepatitis C and HIV co-infection presented for evaluation of an asymptomatic skin rash on the bilateral lower extremities of 6-month duration. The rash appeared as dark brown spots that eventually turned more red. It had been initially diagnosed as lichen planus and treated at an outside institute with triamcinolone 0.1% ointment and clobetasol 0.05% ointment with no improvement.

Review of Systems: No pertinent positives.

Medical/Surgical History: Recent diagnosis of hepatitis C and HIV.

Medications: None.

Family History: No history of skin cancer or any other cancers.

Social History: Long-term male sexual partner.

Physical Examination: Hyperpigmented discrete and coalescing indurated plaques most notable on the left lower extremity (see Figure 5.2.1); Three violaceous indurated plaques on the right upper medial thigh (×1) and left upper lateral thigh (×2); No genital or mucosal lesions; no palpable cervical, axillary or inguinal lymph nodes.

Pathology: Punch biopsy of the left lower extremity plaque (Figure 5.2.2): (A) Infiltrative vascular proliferation filling the dermis (H&E, 100×); (B) higher power revealing round and slit-like vascular channels (H&E, 200×); and (C) positive nuclear staining of tumor cells for human herpesvirus 8 (200×); consistent with: KS, plaque stage.

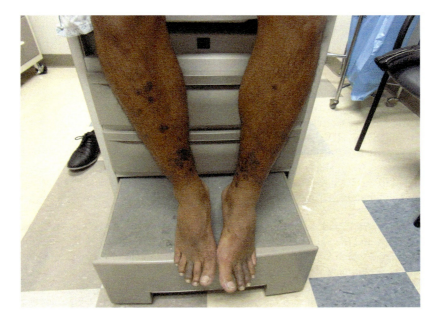

FIGURE 5.2.1 Bilateral lower extremities with hyperpigmented-violaceous indurated plaques.

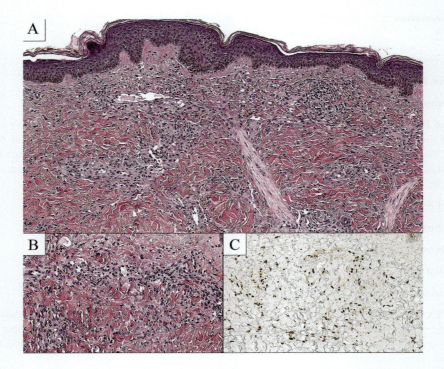

FIGURE 5.2.2   Punch biopsy of a left lower extremity plaque: (A) H&E, 100×; (B) H&E, 200×; and (C) positive nuclear staining of tumor cells for human herpesvirus 8.

Investigations

- **PET/CT skull to thighs:** No evidence of visceral or lymphatic involvement with KS.
- **CD4 count:** 27.
- **HIV viral load:** 22,688 copies/mL.

Final Diagnosis

- KS secondary to HIV infection.

Management and Disease Course: The patient had developed KS without systemic involvement, in the setting of newly diagnosed HIV. He was not yet on any treatment regimen for HIV.

The case was discussed at the multidisciplinary cutaneous oncology tumor board meeting. Antiretroviral therapy (ART) alone was recommended, with a plan to add PLD if the disease progressed or did not respond to ART alone. The patient was started on ART with dolutegravir 50 mg and emtricitabine-tenofovir alafenamide 25 mg daily. He also completed a course of Epclusa for his active hepatitis C infection.

After 2 months of ART, and despite improvement in the white blood cell indices, the KS lesions continued to progress and the patient developed generalized palpable lymphadenopathy. PLD 20 mg/m^2 q3 weeks was initiated which led to an initial clinical response soon after the first infusion. The patient achieved complete resolution of the KS lesions with residual post-inflammatory hyperpigmentation after six cycles of PLD. The chemotherapy was stopped, and the patient was maintained on ART alone. He remained in complete remission until 6 months after discontinuation of PLD. He then developed local recurrence of KS at the right thigh region, which resolved with the application of topical imiquimod five times weekly for 3 months.

Discussion

- Although some patients with epidemic KS see improvement or complete resolution with the initiation of ART alone, such therapy is not sufficient in others. In these cases, liposomal doxorubicin can be utilized to aid in complete clearance of KS lesions, as demonstrated in this case.
- At the height of the AIDS epidemic in the United States during the 1990s, KS became highly associated with the immunosuppression experienced with HIV infection. HIV-positive patients had a 50,000-fold increased risk of developing KS compared to the general population in the pre-ART era. KS was officially declared an AIDS-defining cancer in 1993 by the Centers for Disease Control and Prevention.[1]
- With the development of ART, several studies have documented a 33%–95% decrease in the incidence of this disease. Protease inhibitor-based ART (PI) is speculated to have played an important role in this decline. Use of PI regimens resulted in a 66%–86% response rate and 35% complete remission rate.[2,3] The mechanism for such clinical responses is thought to be multifactorial, including direct anti-angiogenic activity and improvement in the immune response against HHV-8. PIs also inhibit HIV replication and decrease production of the HIV-1 transactivating protein Tat.[2,3]
- Patients on PI may be switched to non-nucleoside reverse transcriptase inhibitor (NNRTI)-based ART. Some studies have reported that such a switch may result in the development of KS, unrelated to the failure of the NNRTI-based ART regimens to control HIV, given that viral loads and CD4 counts remain stable in patients with such recurrences.[2,3] Paparizos et al. showed that switching from a PI to NNRTI-based regimen resulted in an increased risk of developing KS for the first time or having a recurrence of pre-existing KS. Among 724 patients who remained on a PI-based regimen, none developed new KS or had a recurrence. Among 604 patients that switched to an NNRTI-based regimen, four (0.7%) developed KS for the first time. Of the 17 who had a pre-existing KS history whose regimens were switched, three (17.6%) had a recurrence of KS.[3] In contrast, other studies such as the Chelsea and Westminster cohort have shown no difference in the development of KS in patients on PI versus NNRTI-based ART regimens.[2]
- In patients who have progression of KS despite starting ART, systemic chemotherapeutic agents are initiated. A systematic review comparing studies that looked at ART plus chemotherapy versus ART alone showed a significant reduction in KS progression in the ART plus chemotherapy group, suggesting a combination approach may be more effective.[4]
- In comparing specific chemotherapeutic agents, no difference was noted in disease progression between paclitaxel and PLD or between PLD and liposomal daunorubicin. PLD is preferred over free doxorubicin due to its better end-organ specificity and tolerability. Free doxorubicin is associated with more blistering, nausea/vomiting, cardiotoxicity, and alopecia compared to PLD. Of considerable importance, liposomal anthracyclines such as PLD can be given for prolonged periods with very low rates of observed cardiotoxicity, allowing control of recurrent KS in patients over many years. In contrast, free doxorubicin will induce cardiomyopathy when used to high cumulative lifetime dosages (over 400 mg/m^2) and prolonged use of paclitaxel results in disabling neuropathy. For these reasons, PLD is currently considered a generally well-tolerated and safe first-line therapy for KS patients that require systemic chemotherapy.

Teaching Pearls

- Initiation of ART in patients with AIDS-associated KS can completely resolve KS and should be first-line treatment.
- The addition of chemotherapeutic agents to ART may be beneficial for KS patients, particularly those who progress despite ART. Liposomal-encapsulated anthracyclines such as PLD are typically well-tolerated and effective in such patients.

References

1. Ji Y, Lu H. Malignancies in HIV-infected and AIDS patients. *Adv Exp Med Biol*. 2017;1018:167–179.
2. La Ferla L, Pinzone M, Nunnari G, et al. Kaposi's sarcoma in HIV-positive patients: the state of art in the HAART-era. *Eur Rev Med Pharmacol Sci*. 2013;17(17):2354–2365.
3. Paparizos V, Kyriakis K, Kourkounti S, et al. The influence of a HAART regimen on the expression of HIV-associated Kaposi sarcoma. *J Acquir Immune Defic Syndr*. 2008;49(1):111.
4. Gbabe O, Okwundu C, Dedicoat M, et al. Treatment of severe or progressive Kaposi's sarcoma in HIV-infected adults. *Cochrane Database Syst Rev*. 2014;(9):CD003256.
5. Gabizon A, Patil Y, La-Beck N. New insights and evolving role of pegylated liposomal doxorubicin in cancer therapy. *Drug Resist Updat*. 2016;(29):90–106.

Case 5.3

Authors: Nicole Patzelt, Sara Al Janahi, Iman Fatima Khan, and Debjani Sahni.

Reason for Presentation: A case of non-epidemic KS.

Chief Complaint: New rash on the left leg.

History of Present Illness: A young patient with male to female gender reassignment, presented for management of newly diagnosed KS. Two months prior to presentation, she had developed two asymptomatic, well-defined, reddish-purple patches on the left popliteal fossa and left lower ankle, associated with painful left leg swelling. They had not enlarged since they first appeared. The lesions had been biopsied and confirmed as KS by a dermatologist from an outside institute. A prior recent HIV test was negative. The patient was a transgender woman who had sexual intercourse with men. Although she denied a history of long-term immunosuppression, she had poorly controlled atopic dermatitis that had been previously treated with 2–3 courses of oral prednisone (usually 25 mg tapers) per year for the past few years.

Review of Systems: No pertinent positives.

Medical/Surgical History: Gender reassignment surgery, atopic dermatitis previously treated with frequent courses of oral prednisone.

Medications: Nil other than topical steroids.

Family History: No family history of skin cancer.

Social History: Nil relevant.

Physical Examination: Left popliteal fossa with a 3×4 mm well-defined indurated violaceous thin plaque (see Figure 5.3.1); surrounding the left malleolus were three violaceous shiny papules; left leg with non-pitting edema; small, mobile palpable left axillary lymphadenopathy <0.5 cm.

Pathology: Punch biopsy of the left popliteal fossa plaque (see Figure 5.3.2): (a) A superficial and deep interstitial tumor with perivascular inflammation (H&E, 40×); (b) Spindle cells and slit-like vascular channels dissecting between collagen bundles partly surrounding pre-existing blood vessels (promontory sign) (H&E, 100×); and (c) Positive nuclear staining of tumor cells for human herpesvirus 8 (100×); consistent with: KS, plaque stage.

Investigations

- PET/CT whole body: No evidence of visceral or lymphatic involvement by KS.
- A repeat HIV test >3 months after the prior one: Still negative.

Final Diagnosis: Kaposi sarcoma that best fits with non-epidemic KS subtype.

Management and Disease Course: Given the localized nature of the KS, topical therapy with imiquimod 5% cream three times per week was initially started. On follow-up, the KS was noted to be progressing and the patient reported new lesions and further swelling on the bilateral lower extremities. Her treatment was reviewed at the cutaneous oncology tumor board. Radiotherapy was deemed impractical as there were multiple scattered lesions on both lower extremities. Consequently, the patient was started on PLD at 20 mg/m^2 every 4 weeks, and was instructed to wear compression stockings and elevate the legs. Improvement was noted soon after the second cycle of PLD with shrinkage of the skin lesions and resolution of the swelling. The patient was noted to develop new-onset pigmented macules on the dorsal hands, as well as hand-foot syndrome as a side effect of the chemotherapy. The latter settled after the fifth cycle of PLD. The patient completed a total of nine cycles of PLD, with complete skin clearance and remains off therapy with no evidence of disease recurrence to date more than 5 years later.

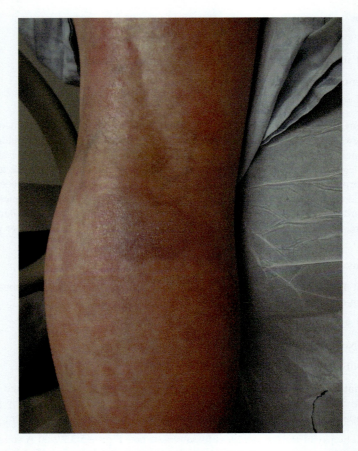

FIGURE 5.3.1   Irregular violaceous plaque in the left popliteal fossa. Note the surrounding eczematous rash.

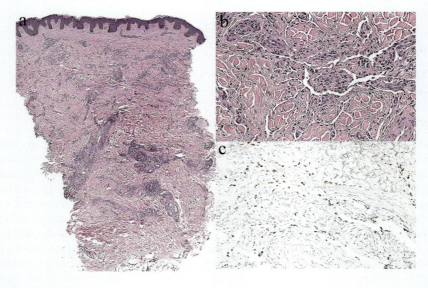

FIGURE 5.3.2   Punch biopsy of a left lower extremity plaque: (a) H&E, 40×; (b) H&E, 100×; and (c) positive nuclear staining of tumor cells for human herpesvirus 8.

Discussion

- KS has been classified historically into four histologically indistinguishable categories: Classic, African-endemic, epidemic (or AIDS-associated), and iatrogenic. Not all patients with KS fit into one of these traditional categories. "Non-epidemic" KS is a relatively recently described subtype of KS, which is seen in MSM, but do not themselves have HIV infection. Our case fits best with this.

- Non-epidemic KS appears to present like classical KS clinically, however, typically affects younger patients (mean age 53 years). Although patients in a series of 28 MSM tended to have a good prognosis with overall limited disease, it is notable that three of the patients in this series went on to develop lymphoproliferative disorders (multicentric Castleman disease, follicular lymphoma and Burkitt's lymphoma). Larger studies are needed to understand the true prognosis of non-epidemic KS.[1]

- HHV-8 is responsible for causing all forms of KS. The virus establishes lifelong latent infection in the host with intermittent periods of viral shedding. The oropharynx is the most common mucosal site for both the replication and transmission of the virus. Practices that lead to exposure to saliva correlate with the acquisition of the virus. The prevalence of HHV-8 varies geographically and is most common in Uganda and Sub-Saharan Africa where >60% of the adult population may be infected. Studies in the United States have been able to demonstrate frequent and intermittent viral shedding from the saliva of immunocompetent MSM. The predilection in MSM may be attributed to the prevalence of oral sexual activity.[2,3]

- Our patient had received multiple courses of oral corticosteroids in the past for poorly controlled atopic dermatitis. The periods of intermittent immunosuppression could have further contributed to the development of KS. Another important component of our patient's treatment was to get the atopic dermatitis under better control so as not to require systemic corticosteroids. This was eventually achieved by instituting tacrolimus 0.1% ointment and good skin care.

- Our patient required PLD to achieve disease control. One of the cutaneous side effects which she developed, and is reported to occur with doxorubicin therapy, is dyspigmentation of the skin and nails. Hyperpigmentation of the skin can be localized or generalized. In the nails, the nail matrix melanocytes are activated by doxorubicin leading to brown-black to blue-black pigmentation. The pigmentation is typically reversible within 1–2 months of discontinuing doxorubicin.[4] One series found 21% of their 64 patients developed hyperpigmentation while on doxorubicin therapy. Four of those patients had total body hyperpigmentation.[5]

Teaching Pearls

- KS has traditionally been subdivided into four categories: Classic, endemic, epidemic (AIDS-associated), and iatrogenic.
- "Non-epidemic" KS is a relatively new subtype that develops in young MSM without overt evidence of immunodeficiency. The data reported so far suggests an overall good prognosis, though evidence from larger studies is needed to corroborate this.
- Treatment with doxorubicin can cause skin and nail dyspigmentation that is generally reversible with discontinuation of therapy.

References

1. Lanternier F, Lebbe C, Schartz N, et al. Kaposi's sarcoma in HIV-negative men having sex with men. *AIDS*. 2008;22(10):1163–1168.
2. Casper C, Krantz E, et al. Frequent and asymptomatic oropharyngeal shedding of human herpesvirus 8 among immunocompetent men. *J Infect Dis*. 2007;195(1):30–36.
3. Ignacio R, Goldman J et al. Patterns of human herpesvirus-8 oral shedding among diverse cohorts of human herpesvirus-8 seropositive persons. *Infect Agent Cancer*. 2016;11:7.
4. Maiti A, Bhattacharya S. A patient with cancer and nail pigmentation. *BMJ*. 2016;3:353:i2346.
5. Alagaratnam T, Choi T, Ong G. Doxorubicin and hyperpigmentation. *Aust N Z J Surg*. 1982;52(5):531–533.

Case 5.4

Authors: Bilal Fawaz and Debjani Sahni.

Reason for Presentation: Treatment of refractory KS with pomalidomide.

History of Present Illness: A middle-aged patient with type VI skin presented with a 1-year history of asymptomatic growths and discoloration on the bilateral lower extremities. The patient had accompanying swelling of the bilateral lower extremities but denied any associated pain, bleeding, or itching.

Review of Systems: No pertinent positives.

Relevant Medical and Surgical History: HIV-positive; prior lower leg deep vein thrombosis.

Medications: Bictegravir, emtricitabine, tenofovir, alafenamide, and apixaban.

Family History: No pertinent positives.

Physical Examination: Numerous ill-defined hyperpigmented macules and papules coalescing into large, indurated plaques and nodules scattered throughout the thighs and legs (see Figure 5.4.1); Mild *peau d'orange* appearance along the anteromedial thighs; inguinal adenopathy.

Pathology: Punch biopsy of the left lower leg: Interlacing short fascicles of spindle cells with slit-like blood vessels and scattered erythrocytes. Immunostains for HHV-8 showed positive nuclear stain in tumor cells. The staining was also positive for CD31 but negative for CD34. The morphology and immunoprofile support the diagnosis of KS.

Investigations

- **CD4 count:** 169.
- **Whole-body PET/CT:** Inguinal adenopathy and secondary lymphedema of the lower extremities.

Diagnosis: AIDS-associated KS.

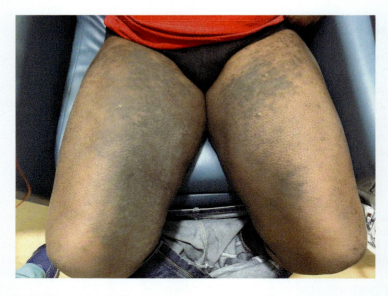

FIGURE 5.4.1 Multiple hyperpigmented dermal papules coalescing into indurated plaques on the bilateral thighs with edema and *peau d'orange* appearance of the surrounding skin.

Management

Given the PET/CT findings, the patient was started on PLD (20 mg/m^2 IV every 3 weeks), with initial improvement in his nodal and cutaneous disease. After 15 months of therapy, the patient experienced disease progression while on liposomal doxorubicin and was therefore switched to paclitaxel 135 mg/m^2 IV every 3 weeks. Unfortunately, the KS progressed after two cycles of paclitaxel and the patient developed peripheral neuropathy, requiring a dose reduction. Pembrolizumab was also added at this point. The combination of paclitaxel and pembrolizumab yielded little benefit after five and three cycles, respectively.

The patient was subsequently switched from paclitaxel to pomalidomide (4 mg orally daily for 21 days/28 day cycle), resulting in an immediate and dramatic clinical response and near-resolution of his cutaneous disease. His disease remains well-controlled to date, more than 12 months after initiation of pomalidomide and pembrolizumab therapy.

Discussion

- Since the initial report of epidemic (AIDS-associated) KS in 1982, the incidence of epidemic KS has dramatically increased in the United States and globally.[1,2] KS is often the first AIDS-defining illness diagnosed in MSM.[1] The introduction of HAART has slowed the rising incidence of KS, but it remains the most common neoplasm diagnosed in HIV patients and a significant public health concern.[1]

- The clinical presentation of KS is highly variable, ranging from a solitary papule or nodule to disseminated cutaneous disease. While the lower extremities and face are commonly involved, lesions may arise anywhere on the body.[1] Individuals classically present with oval-round, violaceous-brown patches, plaques, and nodules, although findings can be subtle, arising as faint erythematous or hyperpigmented macules and patches.[1] Intra-oral involvement is common, and visceral disease may be present, most frequently involving the gastrointestinal tract, lymph nodes, and lungs.[1]

- No universally accepted staging system currently exists for KS. The National Institute of Health's AIDS Clinical Trial Group (ACTG) remains the most commonly used staging system, although this is typically utilized in a research setting.[2] The ACTG system categorizes patients based on three criteria: (a) Extent of tumor (T; with extensive oral cavity involvement or visceral disease considered poor prognostic signs); (b) immune status (I; CD4+ count <200 cells/μL considered a poor prognostic sign); and (c) severity of systemic illness (S; history opportunistic infection, thrush, fevers, night sweats, weight loss, diarrhea >2 weeks considered poor prognostic signs).[2]

- A more recent prognostic index has been proposed by Stebbing et al. based on the following four criteria: KS as the AIDS-defining illness; age of 50 years or older; low CD-4+ count; and presence of a concurrent AIDS-associated illness.[1] Authors recommend that patients with a score >12/15 should be initially treated with HAART and systemic chemotherapy, whereas treatment should be limited to HAART alone in patients with a score <5/15.[1]

- The staging systems should be used to guide therapeutic decisions in a case-dependent manner. The mainstay of therapy for epidemic KS is HAART, and its importance should be stressed to patients.[3] The addition of skin-directed therapies may be considered in patients with localized disease.[3] Topical alitretinoin 0.1% gel and imiquimod 5% cream have achieved favorable responses in some cases for limited cutaneous disease. Intra-lesional chemotherapy, cryotherapy, laser treatment, photodynamic therapy, and excisional surgery may also be considered.[3] Radiotherapy represents an excellent option in patients with localized disease, with reported response rates as high as 91%.[3]

- In the presence of poor prognostic features, systemic chemotherapy should be considered. Typical indications include extensive cutaneous (>20) or oral cavity involvement, symptomatic pedal or scrotal edema, symptomatic visceral involvement, and flare due to immune reconstitution inflammatory syndrome.[1,2] Liposomal doxorubicin, liposomal daunorubicin, and paclitaxel are typically the chemotherapeutic agents of choice.[3] A recent Cochrane review concluded that in severe or progressive disease, the addition of systemic chemotherapy to HAART may be beneficial in reducing disease progression in AIDS-associated KS.[3]

- In cases where patients progress despite liposomal anthracyclines and paclitaxel, pomalidomide is an emerging therapeutic option for symptomatic KS.[4] Pomalidomide is an oral thalidomide derivative with antiproliferative and immunomodulatory properties. The mechanism of action involves targeting an E3 ubiquitin ligase (cereblon), leading to enhancement of CD4+ and CD8+ T-cell co-stimulation.[4]

- A recent phase II clinical trial investigating pomalidomide's efficacy for KS demonstrated a response rate of 60% among HIV-positive patients, with 100% response rate in HIV-negative patients.[4] Patients were treated with 5 mg daily for 21 days per 28-day cycle, with a dose reduction to 3 mg if not tolerated (median of seven cycles; range 2–12).[4] Treatment was continued for a maximum of 1 year or until patients developed complete response, progression, or intolerable adverse events. The main grade 3 adverse events were neutropenia (ten patients, 23 cycles), infection (one patient), and edema (one patient).[4] The authors also noted that responses were rapid, with a median time of 4 weeks.[4]

- PD-1 inhibitors, such as pembrolizumab and nivolumab, are also emerging as a viable treatment option for advanced, refractory KS.[5] While evidence remains limited to retrospective studies and case reports, a recent systematic review concluded that PD-1 inhibitors may be safe and effective in HIV patients.[5] Among eight patients with AIDS-associated KS treated with nivolumab, one achieved complete remission, four achieved partial remissions, and three demonstrated disease progression, for an overall response rate of 63%.[5] The PD-1 inhibitors were well-tolerated, and the HIV remained suppressed in 93% of cases.[5] Several ongoing clinical trials are further investigating the safety and efficacy of immune checkpoint inhibitors for HIV-associated malignancies.[5]

Teaching Pearls

- Although no universally accepted staging systems exist, the ACTG staging system and the prognostic index proposed by Stebbing et al. can help guide management for patients with epidemic KS.

- The mainstay of therapy for epidemic KS is HAART.

- Systemic chemotherapy with liposomal anthracyclines and paclitaxel should be considered in select patients especially individuals with the following risk factors: Extensive cutaneous, oral, or symptomatic visceral disease; CD4+ count <200 cells/μL; other concurrent AIDS-defining illnesses; or advanced age (>50 years).

- Pomalidomide and PD-1 inhibitors may be considered in refractory disease where patients have failed treatment with HAART and first-line chemotherapy drugs.

References

1. Stebbing J, Sanitt A, Nelson M, et al. A prognostic index for AIDS-associated Kaposi's sarcoma in the era of highly active antiretroviral therapy. *Lancet.* 2006;367(9521):1495–1502.
2. Krown SE, Metroka C, Wernz JC. Kaposi's sarcoma in the acquired immune deficiency syndrome: a proposal for uniform evaluation, response, and staging criteria. AIDS Clinical Trials Group Oncology Committee. *J Clin Oncol.* 1989;7(9):1201–1207.
3. Gbabe OF, Okwundu CI, Dedicoat M, et al. Treatment of severe or progressive Kaposi's sarcoma in HIV-infected adults. *Cochrane Database Syst Rev.* 2014 ;(9):CD003256. doi:10.1002/14651858.CD003256.pub2.
4. Polizzotto MN, Uldrick TS, Wyvill KM, et al. Pomalidomide for symptomatic Kaposi's sarcoma in people with and without HIV infection: a phase I/II study. *Clin Oncol.* 2016;34(34):4125–4131.
5. Cook MR, Kim C. Safety and efficacy of immune checkpoint inhibitor therapy in patients with HIV infection and advanced-stage cancer: a systematic review. *JAMA Oncol.* 2019;5(7):1049–1054.

6

Dermatofibrosarcoma Protuberans

Bilal Fawaz and Debjani Sahni

CONTENTS

Introduction

Dermatofibrosarcoma protuberans (DFSP) is a rare fibroblastic neoplasm characterized by slow, relentless growth and a low metastasis rate.[1] DFSP accounts for 0.1% of all malignancies and has an estimated annual incidence of 4.2 per million in the United States.[2] The tumor can arise at any age but most often develops in the fourth to fifth decades of life.[2] No clear sexual predilection exists as studies have been mixed.[1–3] African Americans are known to have a higher risk of developing the neoplasm, with one study reporting almost double the risk in blacks compared to other races.[2]

DFSP most commonly develops on the trunk as a pink-brown, indurated papule, slowly expanding into its characteristic firm, multinodular presentation.[3] Overlying atrophy, ulceration, and/or hyperkeratosis may be present.[2] The trunk is the most common location (42% of cases), followed by the upper extremities (23%), lower extremities (18%), and the head and neck region (16%).[2] The insidious, largely asymptomatic presentation of the tumor often leads to a delay in diagnosis, resulting in significant subclinical extension and large size on presentation.[2–4] The differential diagnosis of skin lesions with this appearance also contributes to delay in diagnosis as it includes numerous benign entities such as keloids, vascular malformations, dermatofibromas, and dermal dendrocyte hamartomas, among others.[2]

Histologically, a dermal proliferation of spindled fibroblasts arranged in a storiform or fascicular pattern is typically present.[5] The cells infiltrate collagen bundles and extend into underlying subcutaneous tissue in a characteristic "honeycomb" pattern.[5] Hyperchromatic nuclei and mitoses are present in advanced disease. The fibrosarcomatous variant has increased cellularity with fascicles arranged in a herringbone pattern.[5] A pigmented variant also exists (i.e., Bednar tumor) characterized by the presence of melanin-producing spindled cells.[6] Immunohistochemically, DFSP is CD34(+) and factor XIIIa(−), whereas benign entities such as dermatofibroma (DF) are typically negative for CD34.[5]

Constitutive over-expression of the *platelet-derived growth factor B* (*PDGFB*) gene on chromosome 22 is believed to play a key role in the development of DFSP. The uncontrolled production *PDGFB* occurs due to a translocation resulting in the fusion of two genes; the *COL1A1* gene located on chromosome 17q22, which encodes the α1 chain of type 1 collagen, and the *PDGFB* gene located on chromosome 22q13, which encodes the β chain of the PDGF ligand. The PDGF receptor, PDGF-R, is a transmembrane tyrosine kinase that is normally expressed by fibroblasts, which upon binding the cytokine PDGFB induces fibroblast cellular proliferation and connective tissue growth. The translocation places the *PDGFB* gene under direct control of the *COL1A1* gene, resulting in its deregulation. The fusion gene product is cleaved

DOI: 10.1201/9780429026683-6

intracellularly into mature *PDGFB*, followed by secretion of this cytokine and autocrine stimulation of tumor growth. A (17;22)(q22;q13) translocation resulting in a collagen1α1 (*COL1A1*)/*PDGFB* fusion gene and resultant growth factor has been identified in up to 90% of DFSP cases, with various other combinations of genetic alterations found in rare cases.[7]

Once the histologic diagnosis is confirmed, imaging should be considered in recurrent or large tumors to better assess the extent of tumor infiltration.[1,8] Contrast magnetic resonance imaging (MRI) is the imaging modality of choice due to its superior ability to detect subcutaneous extension.[8]

Surgical therapy remains first line, either by Mohs micrographic surgery (MMS) or wide local excision (WLE) with complete margin assessment.[9] The key to prevent disease recurrence is an adequate surgical margin, given the infiltrative nature of the tumor. However, margins can be limited due to the anatomical location of the tumor. Adjuvant radiation should be considered in tumors with close or positive margins.[10] Numerous studies suggest that disease-free survival can be improved with post-operative radiation in DFSP patients.[11] Imatinib, a tyrosine kinase inhibitor, may be considered in patients who are not surgical candidates. A recent systematic review on imatinib for the treatment of DFSP revealed a complete response rate of 5.2%, partial response in 55.2%, stable disease in 27.6%, and disease progression in 9.2%.[12]

Local recurrences are frequent (7.3%–25%) after a median time of 32 months.[1–3] Factors predictive of poor outcomes include the fibrosarcomatous histologic subtype, high mitotic index, increased cellularity, advanced age (>50 years), margins <2 cm, and <1 mm margins to positivity after resection.[3,10] However, overall prognosis is favorable due to its infrequent metastasis, with a reported relative 5-year survival of 99.2%.[2]

References

1. Bogucki B, Neuhaus I, Hurst EA. Dermatofibrosarcoma protuberans: a review of the literature. *Dermatol Surg.* 2012;38(4):537–551.
2. Criscione V, Weinstock M. Descriptive epidemiology of dermatofibrosarcoma protuberans in the United States, 1973 to 2002. *J Am Acad Dermatol.* 2007;56:968–973.
3. Bowne WB, Antonescu CR, Leung DH, et al. Dermatofibrosarcoma protuberans: a clinicopathologic analysis of patients treated and followed at a single institution. *Cancer.* 2000;88(12):2711–2720.
4. Saiag P, Grob JJ, Lebbe C, et al. Diagnosis and treatment of dermatofibrosarcoma protuberans. European consensus-based interdisciplinary guideline. *Eur J Cancer.* 2015;51(17):2604–2608.
5. Llombart B, Sanmartin O, Lopez-Guerrero J, et al. Dermatofibrosarcoma protuberans: clinical, pathological, and genetic (COL1A1-PDGFB) study with therapeutic implications. *Histopathology.* 2009;54:860–872.
6. Ding JA, Hashimoto H, Sugimoto T, et al. Bednar tumor (pigmented dermatofibrosarcoma protuberans). An analysis of six cases. *Acta Pathol Jpn.* 1990;40:744–754.
7. Sandberg A, Bridge J. Updates on the cytogenetics and molecular genetics of bone and soft-tissue tumors: dermatofibrosarcoma protuberans and giant cell fibroblastoma. *Cancer Genet Cytogenet.* 2003;140(1):1–12.
8. Lee S, Mahoney M, Shaughnessy E. Dermatofibrosarcoma protuberans of the breast: imaging features and review of the literature. *Am J Roentgenol.* 2009;193:W64–W69.
9. Durack A, Gran S, Gardiner MD, et al. A 10-year review of surgical management of dermatofibrosarcoma protuberans. *Br J Dermatol.* 2021;184(4):731–739.
10. Dagan R, Morris CG, Zlotecki RA, et al. Radiotherapy in the treatment of dermatofibrosarcoma protuberans. *Am J Clin Oncol.* 2005;28:537–539.
11. Du K, Li J, Tang L, et al. Role of postoperative radiotherapy in dermatofibrosarcoma protuberans: a propensity score-matched analysis. *Radiat Oncol.* 2019;14(1):20.
12. Navarrete-Dechent C, Mori S, Barker CA, et al. Imatinib treatment for locally advanced or metastatic dermatofibrosarcoma protuberans: a systematic review. *JAMA Dermatol.* 2019;155(3):361–369.

Case 6.1

Authors: Ali Al-Haseni, MD, Sarah Phillips, MD, Tatchai Ruangrattanatavorn, MD, MSc, Elizabeth T. Rotrosen, AB, and Teviah E. Sachs, MD.

Reason for Presentation: Surgical approach to DFSP.

Chief Complaint: Bump on the right shoulder.

History of Present Illness: A 43-year-old female presented with a 5-year history of an enlarging bump on her right shoulder. It was previously diagnosed as a keloid at an outside institute, and the lesion had been injected with intralesional triamcinolone acetonide 40 mg/mL without improvement. She also reported recent-onset lesional tenderness as well as restricted range of motion overlying her right shoulder.

Review of Systems: No pertinent positives.

Medical/Surgical History: No personal history of skin cancer.

Medications: None.

Family History: No family history of skin cancer. Uncle with gastric cancer.

Social History: None relevant.

Physical Exam: Right shoulder: well defined, pink to light brown, multinodular, firm tumor (see Figure 6.1.1). The tumor extended subcutaneously beyond the visible margins.

Pathology: Punch biopsy of the right shoulder tumor (see Figure 6.1.2): (A) Diffusely infiltrative dermal and subcutaneous tumor (H&E, 10×); (B) higher power revealing spindled cells in a storiform pattern (H&E, 200×); and (C) tumor cells are positive with immunoperoxidase staining for CD34 (200×).

Final Diagnosis: DFSP.

Management: The case was discussed at the cutaneous oncology tumor board panel, and a WLE with 2–3 cm margin was recommended per the NCCN guidelines. CT chest was negative for

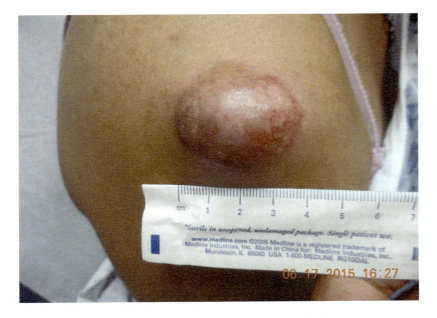

FIGURE 6.1.1 Irregular, multi-lobular, pink, erythematous tumor on the right shoulder.

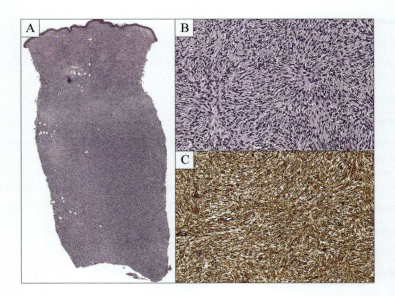

FIGURE 6.1.2 Punch biopsy of the right shoulder tumor: (A) H&E, 10×; (B) H&E, 200×; and (C) positive CD34 immunostain.

metastatic disease. The patient underwent WLE with a 2.5 cm margin, which came back negative on final pathology. Adjuvant radiation was not indicated according to the NCCN guidelines. The patient was monitored closely post-operatively and remained cancer free for the duration of follow-up (5 years) without evidence of local or distant recurrence.

Discussion

- DFSP is a locally aggressive tumor that grows with insidious finger-like projections tracking along subcutaneous fat septae. These projections extend well beyond clinically appreciable tumor, leading to high rates of recurrence and difficulty in achieving clear margins in the operating room. Therefore, excising the tumor down to the level of superficial fascia and achieving negative margins on final pathology is crucial to prevent local recurrence.[1]

- Surgical management is the treatment of choice to clear the tumor, but there is no gold standard approach. There is an ongoing debate as to whether MMS or WLE results in better outcomes.[2]

- Determining adequate margins in both MMS and WLE of DFSP is another area of ongoing research. Various specialties can treat DFSP patients; therefore, different treatment protocols are utilized. Dermatologists tend to prefer MMS, while surgeons (plastic, general, oncological, or head and neck surgeons) prefer WLE.[2–4]

- The data show that achieving negative pathological margins is the key to preventing local recurrence and is more important than the actual choice of surgical approach.[2–4] Additionally, tumors without fibrosarcomatous changes on pathology are believed to have less aggressive biology. They are most likely not capable of metastasizing and can be treated with a more conservative surgical approach. However, the tumor needs to be examined by an experienced pathologist to judge the presence or absence of such changes.[2]

- There are no randomized controlled clinical trials comparing MMS with WLE for DFSP, but there have been several non-randomized comparative studies.[3–5] The most recent data comparing WLE and MMS showed improved tumor clearance and recurrence-free survival in patients treated with MMS. The recurrence with MMS was 3% compared to 30.8% with WLE after a mean follow-up duration of 4.8 and 5.7 years, respectively.[3]

- The current NCCN guidelines (version 1.2021) recommend MMS or other forms of excision with complete circumferential peripheral and deep margin assessment (CCPDMA) as a first-line treatment of DFSP. WLE is recommended when the previous two modalities are unavailable.[6]
- WLE is considered a good treatment option for large tumors in low-risk areas or in tumors with aggressive pathology (fibrosarcomatous changes). It is considered a time and resource-saving treatment modality compared to Mohs.[2,4] However, it can result in significant morbidity in high-risk, cosmetically or functionally sensitive areas due to the need for complex reconstructive techniques (flaps/grafts) to repair the large resection defect. On the other hand, while treating DFSP with MMS is ideal for small tumors in high-risk areas, it needs to be emphasized that Mohs is a highly specialized procedure, done under local anesthesia, and requires trained staff and specific equipment for CD34 staining of frozen sections to confirm negative margins, which may not be available at every institution. Patients may need to travel long distances to reach such specialized centers, making it impractical. Lastly, for relatively small tumors on the trunk or extremities, another option is to offer patients the option of WLE with CCPDMA of the pathology specimen so as not to sacrifice improved tumor clearance. This method, although more cumbersome to the pathologist, has a local recurrence rate comparable to MMS with good cosmetic and functional outcome, yet without the cost and inconvenience associated with MMS.[2,4,5]
- If pursuing WLE of DFSP, the current consensus recommends aiming for 2–3 cm margin when possible, and less aggressive, albeit still negative, margins in cosmetically or functionally sensitive areas.[1,7] If treating with MMS, two layers are typically required, or 1–1.3 cm margins to achieve clearance.[1,3]
- Local recurrence occurs most commonly in those patients whose pathologic margins were <1 mm, or in whom the final margins were positive.[8]

Teaching Pearls

- DFSP is a locally aggressive tumor that requires either MMS, excision with CCPDMA, or WLE to achieve clear margins and lower the risk of recurrence.
- When treating DFSP, it is of critical importance to account for both tumor and patient factors in deciding the best therapeutic strategy.

References

1. Saiag P, Grob JJ, Lebbe C, et al. Diagnosis and treatment of dermatofibrosarcoma protuberans European consensus-based interdisciplinary guideline. *Eur J Cancer.* 2015;51(17):2604–2608. doi:10.1016/j.ejca.2015.06.108.
2. van Houdt WJ. Margins in DFSP reconsidered: primum non nocere. *Ann Surg Oncol.* 2020;27(3):634–636. doi:10.1245/s10434-019-08012-4.
3. Lowe GC, Onajin O, Baum CL, et al. A comparison of Mohs micrographic surgery and wide local excision for treatment of dermatofibrosarcoma protuberans with long-term follow-up: the Mayo Clinic experience. *Dermatol Surg.* 2017;43(1):98–106.
4. Mullen JT. Dermatofibrosarcoma protuberans: wide local excision versus Mohs micrographic surgery. *Surg Oncol Clin N Am.* 2016;25(4):827–839.
5. Zwald FO. Underuse of Mohs micrographic surgery for the treatment of dermatofibrosarcoma protuberans: comment on "efficacy of Mohs micrographic surgery for the treatment of dermatofibrosarcoma protuberans". *Arch Dermatol.* 2012;148(9):1064. doi:10.1001/archdermatol.2012.2685.
6. NCCN Guidelines. Accessed 3.9.2021. https://www.nccn.org/professionals/physician_gls/default.aspx#dfsp.
7. Acosta AE, Velez CS. Dermatofibrosarcoma protuberans. *Curr Treat Options Oncol.* 2017;18(9):56. doi:10.1007/s11864-017-0498-5.
8. Bowne WB, Antonescu CR, Leung DH, et al. Dermatofibrosarcoma protuberans: a clinicopathologic analysis of patients treated and followed at a single institution. *Cancer.* 2000;88(12):2711–2720.

Case 6.2

Authors: Sarah Ann Kam, MD, Malathi Chittireddy, MD, MSc, Hanna E. Mumber, BS, and Teviah E. Sachs, MD.

Reason for Presentation: Use of adjuvant radiation in DFSP.

Chief Complaint: Lump in the left groin.

History of Present Illness: A young patient with a history of hidradenitis suppurativa (HS) presented for evaluation of a firm mass in the left inguinal crease. The mass was first noted by the patient 6 months prior to presentation as a small non-tender bump that enlarged slowly over time. There had been a rapid increase in size, however, in the recent 4 weeks despite treatment with warm compresses. The patient denied any pain in the region. Prior suppurative lesions of HS in this region were typically self-limited and resolved either with or without drainage.

Review of Systems: No pertinent positives other than those described above.

Medical/Surgical History: HS.

Medications: Nil relevant.

Family History: Nil relevant.

Social History: Ten-pack-year history of smoking.

Physical Examination: Left groin: 5 cm exophytic, firm, non-tender, smooth, mobile tumor with a purple-red hue (see Figure 6.2.1).

Pathology: Punch biopsy of the left groin (see Figure 6.2.2): Intermediate power demonstrating oval to spindled cells in a storiform pattern (H&E, 100×).

Investigations

- CT abdomen/pelvis revealed a solitary, heterogeneous, and peripherally enhancing lesion within superficial soft tissues of the left groin measuring up to 6.5 cm, concerning for neoplasm.
- Chest X-ray: No evidence of metastatic disease.

Final Diagnosis: DFSP with no evidence of metastasis.

Management and Disease Course: The NCCN guidelines recommend WLE with wide margins of 2–3 cm for DFSP. However, given the location of the tumor adjacent to the genital area, a multidisciplinary tumor board consensus agreed on 0.5–1 cm margin. The operation was successful and achieved a negative margin of 0.5 cm. Adjuvant radiation was recommended to minimize the chance of local recurrence.

The patient underwent fractionated adjuvant radiation over 6 weeks, with a planned dose of 45 Gy followed by a cone down to 55.8 Gy with a total 31 fractions. Treatment was well tolerated with mild to moderate radiation dermatitis (erythema and moist desquamation). This was treated topically with petrolatum and triamcinolone 0.01% ointment. Patient was lost to follow-up after 2.5 years with no evidence of disease recurrence.

Discussion

- The rarity of DFSP has hindered carrying out randomized controlled trials. There is no level I evidence for the use of adjuvant radiation for close negative margins; however, there is some level III data to suggest a benefit to adjuvant radiation in these patients.

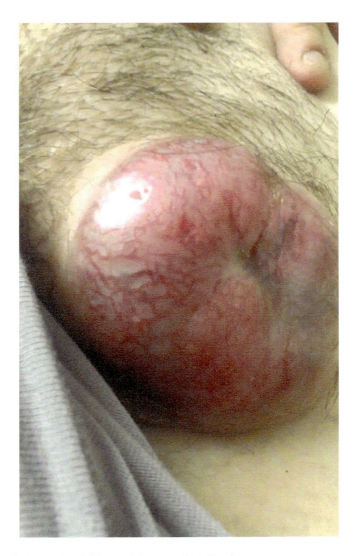

FIGURE 6.2.1 Exophytic, purple-reddish smooth tumor on the left groin.

- Based on the current NCCN guidelines, the recommended first-line treatment for DFSP is surgical therapy, either with MMS or WLE with at least 2 cm margins, in addition to close observation every 6–12 months for at least 5 years.
- DFSP is a locally aggressive tumor with recurrence rates of up to 41%, despite negative margins.[1] Adjuvant radiation therapy is often employed in patients at high risk for recurrence, or those with positive or close margins.[2] The following scenarios are associated with a high risk of recurrence:[2–4]
  - Tumors larger than 5 cm.
  - Recurrent tumors.
  - Tumors with fibro-sarcomatous changes.
  - Tumors in sensitive areas (face, genitalia) where appropriate margins cannot be achieved.
  - Tumors with high Ki-67 expression (≥17%).

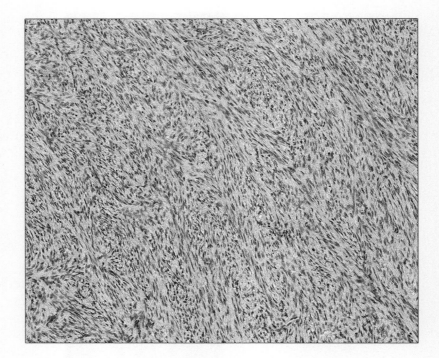

FIGURE 6.2.2   Punch biopsy of the left groin tumor (H&E, 100×).

Teaching Pearls

- DFSP is a rare, soft tissue sarcoma that is often locally aggressive, with recurrence rates as high as 40%, even with negative margins.
- MMS or WLE with 2–3 cm margins is recommended. Sensitive areas may require the use of smaller margins.
- Adjuvant radiation therapy is recommended for all cases with positive margins that cannot be further resected. It may also benefit patients with negative margins who have several high-risk features.

References

1. Lemm D, Mügge L-O, Mentzel T, et al. Current treatment options in dermatofibrosarcoma protuberans. *J Cancer Res Clin Oncol*. 2009;135(5):653–665. doi:10.1007/s00432-009-0550-3.
2. Chen Y-T, Tu W-T, Lee W-R, et al. The efficacy of adjuvant radiotherapy in dermatofibrosarcoma protuberans: a systemic review and meta-analysis. *J Eur Acad Dermatol Venereol*. 2016;30(7):1107–1114. doi:10.1111/jdv.13601.
3. Castle KO, Guadagnolo BA, Tsai CJ, et al. Dermatofibrosarcoma protuberans: long-term outcomes of 53 patients treated with conservative surgery and radiation therapy. *Int J Radiat Oncol Biol Phys*. 2013;86(3):585–590. doi:10.1016/j.ijrobp.2013.02.024.
4. Du K, Li J, Tang L, et al. Role of postoperative radiotherapy in dermatofibrosarcoma protuberans: a propensity score-matched analysis. *Radiat Oncol Lond Engl*. 2019;14(1):20. doi:10.1186/s13014-019-1226-z.

Case 6.3

Authors: Sarah Ann Kam, MD, Sara Al Janahi MD, MSc, Iman Fatima Khan, MS, MPH, and Adam Lerner, MD.

Reason for Presentation: Recurrent, unresectable DFSP treated with a tyrosine kinase inhibitor.

Chief Complaint: Growth on the right shoulder.

History of Present Illness: A young patient with type IV skin presented with a painful, recurrent tumor of the right shoulder. The patient had previously undergone three surgical excisions of tumor masses at this site over a 3-year period. Each excision was followed by tumor recurrence. The patient reported that the current lesion was growing more rapidly than before and causing shoulder pain. The patient was not aware of the tumor type nor did he have copies of his surgical pathology as the operations were performed outside the United States.

Review of Systems: No pertinent positives.

Patient Medical History: None.

Medications: None.

Family History: No pertinent positives.

Physical Examination: A 7.0 × 6.0 cm tender, friable, exophytic tumor with focal necrosis on the right shoulder (see Figure 6.3.1).

Pathology: Punch biopsy of the right shoulder tumor (see Figure 6.3.2): (a) A nodular subcutaneous tumor extending to the inked tissue margin (H&E, 10×) and (b) high power revealing a sheet-like proliferation of uniform plump spindled cells in a myxoid stroma (H&E, 400×).

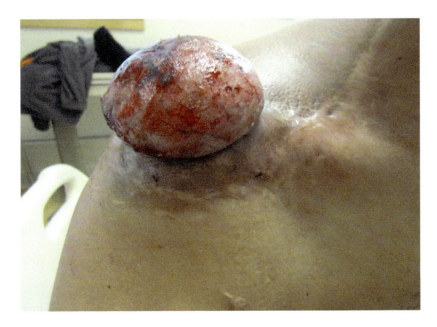

FIGURE 6.3.1 Exophytic friable tumor on the right shoulder.

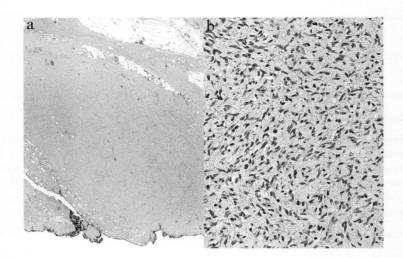

FIGURE 6.3.2   Punch biopsy, right shoulder tumor: (a) H&E, 10× and (b) H&E, 400×.

Investigations

- CT of neck and MRI brachial plexus showed:
- Neoplasm centered around right trapezius with involvement of the paraspinal muscles extending from C3 to T5 and measuring $8 \times 14 \times 13$ cm.

Final Diagnosis: Recurrent and locally advanced DFSP.

Management: At the time of presentation, this was the fourth recurrence of the DFSP on the right shoulder. The multidisciplinary tumor board panel recommended surgical excision with reconstruction followed by adjuvant radiation therapy. The patient underwent radical WLE with extensive soft tissue and muscle resection followed by reconstruction and a split-thickness skin graft from the right thigh. Despite the large excision, his final pathology came back positive for cancer at the lateral and superior margins, and adjuvant radiation was started 6 weeks following the surgery.

A year later after being lost to follow-up, a new mass was detected on examination at the same site of the prior DFSP lesion. Repeat imaging revealed the tumor to be unresectable with invasion to the scapular spine cortex, trapezius and deltoid muscles, and in close proximity to the neurovascular structures of the axilla. As the patient had failed surgery and radiation with subsequent recurrence, the tumor board panel recommended palliative therapy with imatinib 400 mg. While on this medication, the tumor shrunk significantly, and remained stable in size for 1 year of follow-up. The patient did not have significant side effects while on this medication.

Discussion

- DFSP is a cutaneous soft tissue sarcoma that can be locally aggressive. In this case, the patient's tumor recurred four times despite multiple wide local resections. After failing his recent radical surgery and adjuvant radiation therapy, the patient was subsequently started on imatinib, a tyrosine kinase inhibitor (TKI).
- DFSP tumors are frequently responsive to PDGF receptor TKI as the vast majority of them harbor a t(17;22) chromosomal translocation. This leads to the production of a chimeric protein that is proteolytically cleaved within tumor cells, leading to over production of a functional form of PDGF-beta. This cytokine is then secreted, and in an autocrine fashion, binds to and activates tumor PDGF receptors.[1]
- The most widely used TKI is imatinib. The NCCN guidelines recommend imatinib therapy when DFSP tumors are unresectable due to advanced disease, or if resection may lead to significant cosmetic or functional morbidity.

- A systematic review looked at the benefit of imatinib in patients with advanced DFSP who were not surgical candidates due to disease extension that would result in significant cosmetic or functional impairment. Of 152 patients, complete responses were seen in 5.2% cases, partial responses were seen in 55.2% cases, and stable disease was seen in 27.6% of cases. Disease progression was seen in 9.2% of patients.[1] It is notable that risk of progression has been documented to be as high as 45.8% even after a favorable initial response.[2] The use of imatinib in the advanced setting of DFSP is considered palliative.
- Analysis of a systematic review suggests that the efficacy of the lower dose of imatinib (400 mg/day) is similar to the higher dose (800 mg/day) but with more tolerable side effects. It may be better, therefore, to start on a low dose and only increase to higher dosing if no response occurs.[1]
- Guidelines suggest checking for the t(17:22) translocation prior to starting a TKI, though studies have demonstrated efficacy of these drugs even in the absence of the translocation. Further studies are needed to fully understand the utility of genetic testing in selecting treatment and predicting disease response.
- Surgery is the best way to achieve disease cure in DFSP. Imatinib is better utilized in the neoadjuvant setting in DFSP where it can enable surgery to proceed when the tumor is unresectable at presentation. In a systematic review analysis, 60% of patients with initially unresectable disease were able to proceed with surgery following neoadjuvant use of imatinib. Although follow-up data from some of the included studies were limited, results demonstrated a potentially beneficial effect of neoadjuvant imatinib. The majority of patients were documented as being disease-free following surgery, with a reported rate ranging from 60% to 100%.[1] Further studies are needed to assess the duration of response of imatinib in patients with DFSP. Additionally, due to variation in the study methodologies, it is currently not known how long to continue imatinib following surgery. It is also noteworthy that PDGF receptor signaling is important in the early phase of wound healing, as it leads to the recruitment and proliferation of fibroblasts and pericytes. It is important to stop TKIs during the peri-operative period to prevent delayed wound healing and breakdown.[3]
- Other TKIs that have been reported to have activity in the management of advanced DFSP tumors resistant to imatinib include sunitinib and pazopanib (see Table 6.3.1).[3–5]

Teaching Pearls

- Locally advanced and aggressive DFSP that is not amenable to surgery alone can be treated with a TKI, though disease cure is unlikely.
- Imatinib may be utilized in the neoadjuvant setting for locally advanced DFSP. Further studies are needed to define the optimum timing and dosing of imatinib, as well as determining long-term tumor response. It is also important to stop imatinib in the perioperative period to optimize wound healing.

TABLE 6.3.1

Comparison of Tyrosine Kinase Inhibitors in the Treatment of Unresectable DFSP Tumors

Drug	Indication	Dose	Potential Adverse Effects
Imatinib	Unresectable disease	400–800 mg daily	Mucocutaneous eruptions (up to 89%), fever, muscle cramps, GI disturbances, neutropenia, thrombocytopenia. The adverse events are typically mild and tolerable Risk of adverse events correlate with higher dose
Sunitinib	Disease resistant to imatinib	37.5–50 mg daily	Hand-foot syndrome, fatigue, thrombocytopenia, hypertension
Pazopanib	Disease resistant to imatinib	300–400 mg twice daily	Fatigue (65%), GI disturbances, hypertension, hair color changes (38%), mucositis (1%), skin toxicities (<1%)

References

1. Navarrete-Dechent C, Mori S, Barker CA, et al. Imatinib treatment for locally advanced or metastatic dermatofibrosarcoma protuberans: a systematic review. *JAMA Dermatol.* 2019;155(3):361–369. doi:10.1001/jamadermatol.2018.4940.
2. Rutkowski P, Van Glabbeke M, Rankin CJ, et al. European Organisation for Research and Treatment of Cancer Soft Tissue/Bone Sarcoma Group; Southwest Oncology Group. Imatinib mesylate in advanced dermatofibrosarcoma protuberans: pooled analysis of two phase II clinical trials. *J Clin Oncol.* 2010;28(10):1772–1779.
3. Rajkumar VS, Shiwen X, Bostrom M, et al. Platelet-derived growth factor-beta receptor activation is essential for fibroblast and pericyte recruitment during cutaneous wound healing. *Am J Pathol.* 2006;169(6):2254–2265.
4. Fu Y, Kang H, Zhao H, et al. Sunitinib for patients with locally advanced or distantly metastatic dermatofibrosarcoma protuberans but resistant to imatinib. *Int J Clin Exp Med.* 2015;8(5):8288–8294.
5. Xiao W, Que Y, Peng R, et al. A favorable outcome of advanced dermatofibrosarcoma protuberans under treatment with sunitinib after imatinib failure. *OncoTargets Ther.* 2018;11:2439–2443. doi:10.2147/OTT.S150235.
6. Ranieri G, Mammì M, Donato Di Paola E, et al. Pazopanib a tyrosine kinase inhibitor with strong anti-angiogenetic activity: a new treatment for metastatic soft tissue sarcoma. *Crit Rev Oncol Hematol.* 2014;89(2):322–329. doi:10.1016/j.critrevonc.2013.08.012.

7

Merkel Cell Carcinoma

Allene S. Fonseca, Song Park, and Paul Nghiem

CONTENTS

Introduction

Merkel cell carcinoma (MCC) is a rare, aggressive cutaneous malignancy of neuroendocrine origin.[1] Since its initial description by Cyril Toker in 1972, the incidence of MCC has steadily increased, in part due to improved detection.[2–4] A recent estimate in 2011 reported an incidence of 0.79 cases per 100,000 US individuals per year, up from 0.22/100,000 cases/year in 1986.[3] MCC has a strong predilection for elderly, fair-skinned individuals.[3] The mean age at presentation is 74.9 years, most commonly arising in males (61.4%) who are white (94.9%).[3]

Several epidemiological studies have demonstrated a strong association between MCC and ultraviolet (UV) radiation.[3–5] Age-adjusted incidence directly correlates with geographical variations in UVB radiation index, suggesting that UVB exposure plays an integral role in the neoplasm's development.[1,3,5] The discovery of the MC polyomavirus (MCV) and its subsequent detection in the majority of MCC cases provided additional insight into tumor pathogenesis.[6,7] MCV promotes carcinogenesis via various mechanisms, including immune evasion and induction of cellular proliferation.[7] Studies comparing the mutational burden in MCV-negative versus MCV-positive tumors have shown a markedly lower number of mutations in MCV-positive tumors.[8] The results suggest that MCV has potent oncogenic mechanisms that potentiate MCC development in >80% of cases.[6–8]

Clinical findings in MCC are relatively non-specific. The neoplasm presents as a pink-violaceous, erythematous, indurated nodule, often with associated tenderness and rapid growth.[1] The neoplasm arises on the head and neck in the majority of patients >65 years of age, whereas it favors the trunk in younger individuals.[3] Mucosal and metastatic MCCs with no known primary are exceedingly rare but have been reported.[9,10] Histologic features include sheets of small, round, basaloid cells with a "salt and pepper" chromatin pattern and numerous mitotic figures.[11] Positive staining with cytokeratin-20 (CK-20) and neurofilament supports the diagnosis, whereas negative staining with thyroid transcription factor-1 (TTF-1) is essential to rule out metastatic small cell lung carcinoma.[11] CK-7 is generally negative but can be positive in a minority of cases.[11]

MCC displays an aggressive clinical behavior, with high rates of local recurrence and nodal metastasis.[1,3] Therefore, the NCCN guidelines recommend a comprehensive staging evaluation after the diagnosis is established.[12] Evaluation of lymph node disease status is the first step, either via sentinel lymph node biopsy (SLNB) (in the absence of clinically palpable lymphadenopathy) or fine-needle

DOI: 10.1201/9780429026683-7

aspiration versus core biopsy (in the presence of palpable lymphadenopathy).[12] Imaging should also be considered, via MRI, CT, or PET/CT, when there is concern for distant spread.[12]

Surgical management remains first line, with Mohs micrographic surgery or wide local excision (WLE) with 1–2 cm margins.[13] Adjuvant radiation should be considered as it may lower local recurrence rates, although its impact on overall survival remains unclear.[13] Immunotherapy in the setting of advanced disease is promising, but further investigations are warranted. Prognosis remains poor despite therapeutic advances.[1,3,13] The overall 5-year survival rate is 51% for local disease, 35% for nodal disease, and 14% for distant disease.[13] Mortality has paralleled the rising incidence, from 0.03/100,000 persons/ year in 1986 to 0.43/100,000 persons/year in 2011.[3] Close monitoring of patients is therefore recommended, ideally in a multidisciplinary setting, owing to the tumor's highly aggressive clinical behavior.

References

1. Tello TL, Coggshall K, Yom SS, et al. Merkel cell carcinoma: An update and review: Current and future therapy. *J Am Acad Dermatol*. 2018;78(3):445–454.
2. Toker C. Trabecular carcinoma of the skin. *Arch Dermatol*. 1972;105(1):107–110.
3. Fitzgerald T, Dennis S, Kachare S, et al. Dramatic increase in the incidence and mortality from Merkel cell carcinoma in the United States. *Am Surg*. 2015;81:802–806.
4. Agelli M, Clegg LX. Epidemiology of primary Merkel cell carcinoma in the United States. *J Am Acad Dermatol*. 2003;49:832–841.
5. Robertson J, Liang E, Martin R. Epidemiology of Merkel-cell carcinoma in New Zealand: a population-based study. *Br J Dermatol*. 2015;173:835–837.
6. Feng H, Shuda M, Chang Y, et al. 2008 Clonal integration of a polyomavirus in human Merkel cell carcinoma. *Science* 319, 1096–1100.
7. Church CD, Nghiem P. How does the Merkel polyomavirus lead to a lethal cancer? Many answers, many questions, and a new mouse model. *J Invest Dermatol*. 2015;135:1221–1224.
8. Goh G, Waldradt T, Markarov V. Mutational landscape of MCPyV-positive and MCPyV-negative Merkel cell carcinomas 20 with implications for immunotherapy. *Oncotarget*. 2016;7:3403–3415.
9. Yom SS, Rosenthal DI, El Naggar AK, et al. Merkel cell carcinoma of the tongue and head and neck oral mucosal sites. *Oral Surg Oral Med Oral Pathol Oral Radiol Endod*. 2006;101:761–768.
10. Day KE, Carroll WR, Rosenthal EL. Parotid gland metastasis in Merkel cell carcinoma of the head and neck: a series of 14 cases. *Ear Nose Throat J*. 2016;95:398–404.
11. Jour G, Aung PP, Rozas-Muñoz E, et al. Intraepidermal Merkel cell carcinoma: a case series of a rare entity with clinical follow up. *J Cutan Pathol*. 2017;44:684–691.
12. National Comprehensive Cancer Network. Merkel cell carcinoma. Available at: http://merkelcell.org/ wp-content/ uploads/2015/10/MccNccn.pdf. Accessed July, 2020.
13. Harms KL, Healy MA, Nghiem P, et al. Analysis of prognostic factors from 9387 Merkel cell carcinoma cases forms the basis for the new 8th edition AJCC staging system. *Ann Surg Oncol*. 2016;23:3564–3571.

Case 7.1

Authors: Allene S. Fonseca, MD, Song Park, MD, and Paul Nghiem, MD, PhD.

Reason for Presentation: Management of a patient with locoregional MCC by surgery, SLNB, and radiation therapy (RT).

Chief Complaint: Skin lesion.

History of Present Illness: A man in his 50s presented to the dermatology clinic for evaluation of a small firm, red papule on his face medial to his left temple, adjacent to his lateral eyebrow. The lesion was asymptomatic. Over a 10-month period, it grew to approximately 1.5 cm. The lesion was biopsied and confirmed to be MCC. He had had extensive sun exposure since childhood including many outdoor activities. He did not have any profound immunosuppressive conditions.

Review of Systems: No constitutional symptoms. No other new or changing skin lesions on his body.

Patient Medical History: History of a suspected squamous cell carcinoma on his left nasal sidewall 15 years ago.

Medications: Nil relevant.

Family History: Maternal cousin passed away from melanoma at age 40.

Physical Examination: Fair skin complexion with blue eyes and light hair color. Significant sun damage of skin. Approximately 1.5 × 1.0 cm, red, oval, dome-shaped firm nodule medial to the left temple, adjacent to lateral eyebrow (see Figure 7.1.1). No lymphadenopathy of the cervical or axillary lymph nodes.

Histopathology: MCC with strong neuroendocrine marker positivity including CK-20, chromogranin A and synaptophysin (see Figure 7.1.2). Immunohistochemistry (IHC) negative for TTF-1. Margins involved.

Final Diagnosis: MCC of the left temple, pathologic stage I (pT1 pN0 M0; AJCC guidelines Eighth Edition).

Management and Course of Disease

- Baseline PET/CT scan was negative for distant metastatic disease.
- The patient underwent a WLE with SLNB, which revealed zero out of three positive lymph nodes.

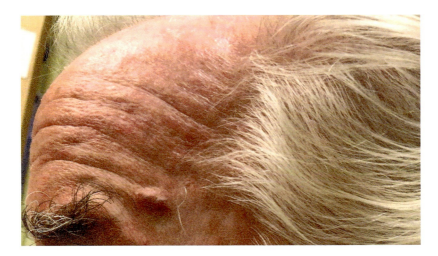

FIGURE 7.1.1 An approximately 1.5 × 1.0 cm, oval, red, dome-shaped firm nodule medial to the left temple, adjacent to lateral eyebrow.

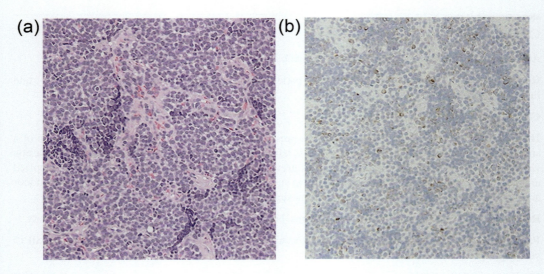

FIGURE 7.1.2   (a) H&E stain of the tumor tissue, demonstrating a poorly differentiated, neuroendocrine carcinoma with characteristic features including basophilic cells with hyperchromatic nuclei and high nuclear to cytoplasmic ratios, which also demonstrate nuclear molding and pronounced mitotic activity (×20 objective), and (b) immunohistochemistry stain demonstrating perinuclear dot-like pattern of CK-20 expression (×20 objective).

- Surgical pathology report of the primary site revealed a 0.6 cm tumor with no lymphovascular invasion (LVI), negative peripheral and deep margins. Distance of carcinoma from the closest peripheral margin was 8 mm.

- He had several low risk factors including the tumor size of 0.6 cm (less than 1 cm), no LVI, widely negative surgical margins, negative SLNB, no immunosuppression. However, he had one high-risk factor of the tumor being located on his head and neck area (see Figure 7.1.3 for detailed risk assessment criteria).

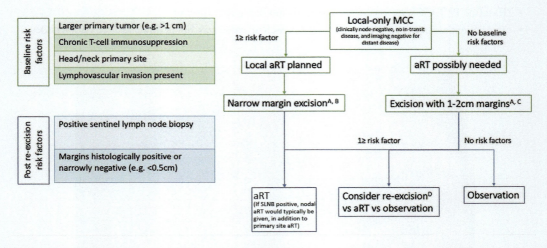

FIGURE 7.1.3   This flowchart integrates treatment options with risk factors that are associated with local recurrence. Certain risk factors are available at the time of diagnosis (baseline), while others are only available after surgical excision (post re-excision). [A] Sentinel lymph node biopsy (SLNB) typically performed at this time; [B] Narrow excision margins minimize morbidity and if aRT is performed microscopically positive margins are acceptable; [C] Goal should be primary tissue closure (i.e., without flap or graft) allowing aRT initiation within 3–4 weeks; [D] Decision on re-excision based on clinical setting (narrow path margins, e.g., <0.5 cm) and patient preference, re-excision vs aRT versus observation. (From Ref. [2] with permission.)

- Based on the risk factor assessment, we decided to give RT to the primary site (46 Gy). The draining node bed was not treated because no lymph nodes were involved according to the SLNB.

Discussion

- MCC is a rare, aggressive malignancy, with high propensity to recur and/or metastasize. Appropriate staging, workup, and initial treatment are essential for optimal management of MCC.
- After the diagnosis of MCC, baseline imaging (e.g., PET/CT) should be carried out, ideally prior to surgery, to determine the extent of disease spread to distant and/or regional sites.
- Upstaging of disease (e.g., a shift from local MCC to regional or distant metastasis) after baseline scan occurs in more than 10% of MCC patients, which is remarkably high compared to melanoma (in which this occurs in less than 1% of cases). Singh et al. analyzed 584 MCC patients with no clinical evidence of distant metastasis who underwent baseline imaging studies. Among patients with non-palpable regional lymph nodes on clinical exam ($n = 492$), 13% were upstaged by imaging and were found to have radiographic nodal involvement or distant metastatic involvement. Among patients with clinically involved regional nodes ($n = 92$), 11% were upstaged to have distant metastatic disease.[1]
- Upstaging information is important because this changes the clinical management and prognosis. It is therefore important to have baseline imaging performed prior to surgery or major decision-making.[1]
- In terms of imaging modality, PET-CT appears to be more sensitive than CT alone at diagnosis for detecting occult metastatic disease.[1]
- Imaging does not replace the need for SLNB in MCC. Nearly one-third of patients had a positive SLNB despite negative imaging and physical examination and were thus upstaged to pathological stage IIIA based solely on their node biopsy data. This procedure thus has both prognostic and therapeutic implications. SLNB should be considered in all patients with no clinical evidence of nodal involvement, who can safely tolerate the procedure.[3]
- In terms of treatment of the primary site, surgical excision and/or RT is the current standard approach. Unlike non-melanoma skin cancers such as squamous or basal cell carcinomas, recurrence beyond a pathologically clear margin is often observed in MCC. However, considering that adjuvant RT (aRT) is often indicated for the primary MCC site, there is controversy over the most appropriate surgical margins to balance morbidity from surgery and to expedite RT.
- To evaluate surgical margin size and recurrence, Tarabadkar et al. analyzed 188 MCC patients presenting with a primary cutaneous MCC tumor and without clinical nodal involvement. They found that if aRT is given, wider surgical margins are not necessary because patients with narrow or even microscopically positive margins have excellent local disease control rate (greater than 98%). The current NCCN guidelines recommend that if aRT is planned, primary closure should be prioritized over wider margins.[2,12].
- Based on the findings from Tarabadkar et al. and the existing literature, Figure 7.1.3 demonstrates a treatment algorithm to aid clinicians in managing primary MCC tumors that integrates risk factors and optimizes local control while minimizing morbidity.[2]
- Obtaining baseline Merkel cell polyomavirus (MCPyV) serology should be considered for prognostic information and surveillance (please refer to Case 7.3 for more information about this test).
- Radiotherapy should often be considered for local control of MCC with the exception of patients who have very low risk disease, as summarized in Figure 7.1.3. If patients have nodal involvement, RT and/or surgery is indicated to the lymph node basin as well.

- For surveillance after treatment, it is important to consider the risk of recurrence depending on the stage. A risk calculator to calculate a given patient's chance (based on stage, sex, immune status, etc.) of experiencing an MCC recurrence is available at https://merkelcell.org/recur. This tool assesses a patient's ongoing risk of recurrence based on the amount of time since initial diagnosis and treatment. Because most recurrences (80%) occur within 2 years of initial diagnosis, a patient's residual risk of recurrence changes rapidly. It is useful to know about the risk of recurrence in determining appropriate surveillance at various timepoints after initial treatment.[3]

Teaching Pearls

- A baseline scan (e.g., PET/CT) is recommended for most patients who are being treated with curative intent. The scan should ideally occur before surgery or finalizing other clinical management decisions.
- If aRT is planned, narrow surgical margins are adequate, reduce morbidity, and minimize delay in initiating radiotherapy.
- The initial treatment modalities for MCC depend on a patient's individual risk and disease extent/stage. SLNB is indicated before WLE. Risk factors that indicate a higher risk of local recurrence (and suggest a need for aRT) include primary tumor location on the head and neck, primary tumor size of >1 cm, chronic immune-suppression, LVI, narrow surgical margins, or positive SLNB.
- Surveillance can be individualized depending on each patient's remaining risk of recurrence over time. https://merkelcell.org/recur.

References

1. Singh N, Alexander NA, Lachance K, et al. Clinical benefit of baseline imaging in Merkel cell carcinoma: analysis of 584 patients. *J Am Acad Dermatol*. 2021 Feb;84(2):330–339.
2. Tarabadkar ES, Fu T, Lachance K, et al. Narrow excision margins are appropriate for Merkel cell carcinoma when combined with adjuvant radiation: analysis of 188 cases of localized disease and proposed management algorithm. *J Am Acad Dermatol*. 2021 Feb;84(2):340–347.
3. Becker JC, Stang A, DeCaprio JA, et al. Merkel cell carcinoma. *Nat Rev Dis Primers*. 2017;3:17077.

Case 7.2

Authors: Allene S. Fonseca, MD, Song Park, MD, and Paul Nghiem, MD, PhD.

Reason for Presentation: Successful treatment of advanced MCC with immunotherapy.

Chief Complaint: Growing lump.

History of Present Illness: A woman in her 60s presented to hospital for edema in her right lower extremity, followed by development of a rapidly growing, painless 3–4 cm lump on her right inguinal area.

Review of Systems: She had recent-onset right leg swelling but did not have significant pain or restriction of activity.

Patient Medical History: History of basal cell carcinoma of the forehead 15–20 years ago; follicular lymphoma in situ which did not need treatment.

Medications: Nil relevant.

Family History: Her mother had breast cancer.

Physical Examination: Two to three palpable lymph nodes in the right inguinal area, each about 3 cm, no other lymphadenopathy; moderate lymphedema of the upper and lower right leg; there were no other papules or nodules to suggest in transit disease.

Histopathology: A 4 cm enlarged lymph node, most consistent with MCC positive for pancytokeratin (AE1/AE3), p63, synaptophysin, p16, and CK-20. IHC negative for MCPyV oncoprotein immunostaining, TTF-1, and S100. No immunophenotypic evidence of lymphoma.

Investigations: Imaging studies demonstrated extensive lymphadenopathy involving the right iliac lymph node chain, and an excisional biopsy confirmed MCC in her right inguinal lymph nodes (see Figure 7.2.1).

Final Diagnosis: Stage IV MCC involving the right inguinal and multiple abdominal lymph nodes with an unknown primary skin lesion.

Management and Course of Disease

- She was a good candidate for immune checkpoint inhibitor treatment without significant co morbidities.
- She was treated with pembrolizumab. Five months later, she had a complete response (CR) to therapy and has remained in CR ever since. She has had surveillance imaging studies every 6 months, which showed no evidence of recurrence of disease. She received a total of 2 years of pembrolizumab. She remains disease-free at the present time, 2 years after her last dose of pembrolizumab.
- She developed type 1 diabetes mellitus approximately 7 months after starting pembrolizumab. Of note, patients who develop an autoimmune complication with cancer immune therapy are modestly more likely to have a favorable anti-cancer response.

Discussion

- SLNB, surgery, or primary RT was not indicated in this patient because she had distant metastatic disease at presentation.
- Prior to the immunotherapy era, the prognosis for stage IV disease was dismal, with a disease-specific survival rate of approximately 15% at 5 years.
- In the past, conventional chemotherapy was the only approach to address advanced MCC. This cancer responds to chemotherapy in approximately 60% of cases. However, responses last for

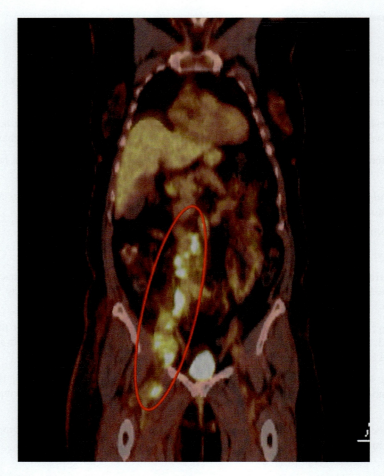

FIGURE 7.2.1   PET-CT demonstrating [^{18}F]-fluorodeoxyglucose (FDG)-avid lymphadenopathy, circled in red, involving right superficial inguinal, ilioinguinal, aortocaval, and retroperitoneal lymph nodes. The largest nodes were up to 4 cm in diameter. In the midline, the bladder has accumulated FDG signal physiologically and the FDG signal background in the liver is also physiologic.

only 90 days on average beyond initiation of chemotherapy. Moreover, prior chemotherapy markedly lowers the likelihood that immunotherapy will work in the future.

- There have been at least three trials investigating the PD-L1 inhibitor avelumab, and PD-1 inhibitors pembrolizumab, and nivolumab in the metastatic setting.[2–4] The response rate in MCC is 50%–70% when those agents are used as first-line treatment and around 30% when given after chemotherapy (in second or later lines of therapy). Therefore, first-line treatment with a PD-L1/PD-1 inhibitor is favored over chemotherapy.

- The response rate was not statistically different between MCPyV-positive or negative MCC across any of the trials.

- Treatment-related adverse events occurred in 68%–96% of patients with ~30% grade 3 or higher adverse events.[1–5] Fatigue was the most common side effect.[2,3] Among grade 3 or higher immune-related adverse events, myocarditis, and transaminitis were commonly reported.[2,3]

- Response is rapid in general, with about 80% of patients having a response in the first 7 weeks.[2]

- Nghiem et al. performed a phase II trial of pembrolizumab in MCC patients who were naïve to systemic therapy. Among the pembrolizumab responders, 80% had responses lasting beyond 2 years.[1]

- These trials demonstrated that PDL-1/PD-1 inhibitors are much more durable and have less toxicity compared to historical data for chemotherapy.[2] Immunotherapy is now listed in the NCCN guidelines for MCC as well as FDA approval for both avelumab (March 2017) and pembrolizumab (December 2018) in the treatment of advanced MCC.

Teaching Pearls

- PD-L1/PD-1 inhibitors are the treatment of choice for metastatic or unresectable MCC in eligible patients.
- The response rate is about 50%–70%. When they occur, responses are typically rapid in onset and durable in the majority of cases.
- While immunotherapy is better tolerated in general than chemotherapy, the majority of patients will experience side effects (fatigue is most common) and a minority will experience significant autoimmune adverse events.
- Because such autoimmune processes can affect almost any tissue or organ system, the patient and clinician must be vigilant to detect and evaluate any significant change in health. Rapidly addressing potentially serious autoimmune complications early is potentially lifesaving by discontinuing immunotherapy and initiating corticosteroids.

References

1. Nghiem P, Bhatia S, Lipson EJ, et al. Durable tumor regression and overall survival in patients with advanced Merkel cell carcinoma receiving pembrolizumab as first-line therapy. *J Clin Oncol.* 2019;37(9):693–702.
2. Kaufman HL, Russell J, Hamid O, et al. Avelumab in patients with chemotherapy-refractory metastatic Merkel cell carcinoma: a multicentre, single-group, open-label, phase 2 trial. *Lancet Oncol.* 2016;17(10):1374–1385.
3. Nghiem PT, Bhatia S, Lipson EJ, et al. PD-1 blockade with pembrolizumab in advanced Merkel-cell carcinoma. *N Engl J Med.* 2016;374(26):2542–2552.
4. Topalian, SL, Bhatia S, Hollebecque A, et al. Abstract CT074: non-comparative, open-label, multiple cohort, phase 1/2 study to evaluate nivolumab (NIVO) in patients with virus-associated tumors (CheckMate 358): efficacy and safety in Merkel cell carcinoma (MCC). *Cancer Research.* 2017;77 (suppl. 13).
5. D'Angelo SP, Russell J, Lebbé C, et al. Efficacy and safety of first-line avelumab treatment in patients with stage iv metastatic Merkel cell carcinoma: a preplanned interim analysis of a clinical trial. *JAMA Oncol.* 2018;4(9): e180077.

Case 7.3

Authors: Allene S. Fonseca, MD, Song Park, MD, and Paul Nghiem, MD, PhD.

Reason for Presentation: Using the MCPyV oncoprotein antibody test to detect MCC recurrence.

Chief Complaint: Growth on the buttocks.

History of Present Illness: A man in his 60s presented with an MCC on the right buttock (1.5 cm). This was treated with excision, SLNB (0/2 nodes were involved; pathologic stage I), and RT to the primary site on the right buttock. We obtained an MCPyV oncoprotein antibody test 1 month after his initial diagnosis, which was positive with a baseline titer of 2,531 (normal <74). He continued to have antibody testing performed every 3 months, and the titer continued to downtrend quickly over the first year after removal of the tumor. Between 9 months and 3 years, his antibody level remained stable between 100 and 200. Three years after his initial diagnosis, his titer increased from 145 to 2,900 over the course of 6 months.

Review of Systems: Nil relevant.

Patient Medical History: History of basal cell carcinomas and hypothyroidism.

Patient Social History: He had Agent Orange exposure while in Vietnam.

Medications: Levothyroxine.

Family History: Daughter had recurrent breast cancer.

Physical Examination (after initial surgery was done, at the time of first MCPyV oncoprotein antibody test): Patient was a fair-skinned individual. A 7 cm horizontal scar below the waistline on the right buttock. No visual or palpable evidence of recurrent disease on the surgery site. No lymphadenopathy in the right inguinal node bed.

Histopathology: Small, round cells with hyperchromatic nuclei and scant cytoplasm, with CK-20 in a dot-like pattern, and TTF1 negative, highly consistent with MCC. There was no LVI, and the margins were negative.

Final Diagnosis: Pathologic stage I MCC on the right buttock. Tumor marker increase at 3 years after initial treatment suggests recurrent disease.

Management and Course of Disease

- Because of the oncoprotein antibody increase, a CT of his chest, abdomen, and pelvis was obtained, which revealed lymphadenopathy in one right inguinal lymph node (see Figure 7.3.1).
- He received one dose of neoadjuvant nivolumab in a clinical trial setting followed by a right inguinal lymph node excision which confirmed MCC. His restaging radiologic study performed just prior to his surgery showed a partial response after one dose of nivolumab.
- Nivolumab was discontinued due to neurological symptoms including diplopia that occurred a week after infusion. This completely resolved by approximately 1 month after discontinuation of immune therapy and initiation of a 4-week course of prednisone. He continues to be followed with MCPyV oncoprotein antibody tests along with scans and has no evidence of disease 4 years after this recurrence.
- In summary, the AMERK test detected his MCC recurrence which was successfully treated with neoadjuvant immunotherapy and surgery.

Discussion

- The majority of MCC tumors (~80% in the United States) are caused by MCPyV. About 50% of MCC patients produce antibodies to the MCPyV oncoprotein (seropositive).

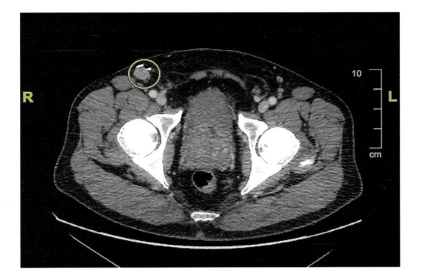

FIGURE 7.3.1 Diagnostic CT with contrast demonstrating an asymmetric, enlarged lymph node (adjacent to the surgical clips), circled in yellow, measuring 1.9 × 1.3 cm, enlarged from 1.0 × 0.8 cm 2 years prior.

- Patients who have undetectable antibody levels at the time of MCC diagnosis (seronegative) are 42% more likely to have a recurrence than those who are seropositive.[3] Thus, patients who are seronegative should be followed with regular imaging studies, and patients who are seropositive should have their oncoprotein antibody titers tracked every 3–4 months, while they remain at significant risk of recurrence.[1]

- Therefore, determining the baseline titer of MCPyV oncoprotein antibodies is useful for initial workup of all patients as it helps to guide their subsequent surveillance.

- An increasing level of MCPyV antibodies has a positive predictive value of 99% for disease recurrence, whereas a significantly decreasing titer has a negative predictive value of 99%.[3] If a patient has an increasing antibody titer, obtaining imaging studies to locate a possible recurrence should be considered, as we did with the patient in this case (see Figure 7.3.2).

- Because the test is highly sensitive, at the time of antibody increase, about 10% of patients will not yet manifest clinically evident disease. These patients should be followed closely for possible recurrent disease. Assuming the antibody titer continues to increase, it is highly likely they will subsequently develop clinically evident disease within the next 6–12 months.[5]

- For patients who are seropositive, this blood test spares them the contrast dye and radiation exposure associated with having multiple scans. It is also less costly, more sensitive, and specific.[1] For these reasons, the NCCN guidelines have listed this test as part of the algorithm for MCC workup since 2018.

Teaching Pearls

- Consider obtaining MCPyV oncoprotein antibody test within 3 months of the initial diagnosis. For seropositive patients, repeat the test every 3–4 months thereafter until the residual risk of recurrence is less than 2%.

- A significant increase in titer has a high positive predictive value and should prompt appropriate imaging studies to locate possible metastatic disease.

- A decreasing or negative titer has a high negative predictive value that the patient is not experiencing a recurrence.

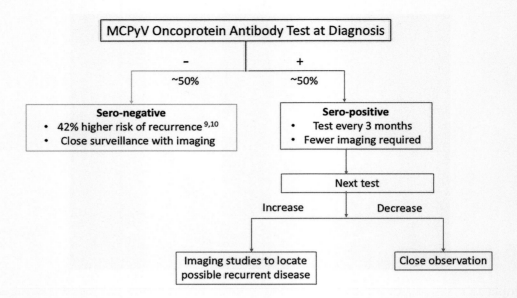

FIGURE 7.3.2   This flowchart illustrates the MCPyV oncoprotein antibody (AMERK) test. The AMERK test should first be obtained at initial diagnosis. About 50% of patients with MCC will produce antibodies to the MCPyV oncoprotein (seropositive). If a patient is seropositive, this test can be repeated every 3 months as a surveillance method. If the AMERK test reveals a significant rise in the antibody titer, imaging studies should be considered to locate possible recurrent disease. If the AMERK test reveals a decrease in the antibody titer, this indicates that the patient's MCC tumor burden is decreasing or no clinical evidence of recurrent disease. If the AMERK test is negative (seronegative), patient should be followed with imaging studies for surveillance because patients who are seronegative have a 42% higher risk of recurrence.

References

1. Paulson KG, Lewis CW, Redman MW, et al. Viral oncoprotein antibodies as a marker for recurrence of Merkel cell carcinoma: a prospective validation study. *Cancer*. 2017;123(8):1464–1474.
2. Paulson KG, Carter JJ, Johnson LG, et al. Antibodies to Merkel cell polyomavirus T antigen oncoproteins reflect tumor burden in Merkel cell carcinoma patients. *Cancer Res*. 2010;70(21):8388–8397.
3. Nghiem P, Park SY. Less toxic, more effective treatment—a win-win for patients with Merkel cell carcinoma. *JAMA Dermatol*. 2019;155(11):1223–1224.
4. National Comprehensive Cancer Network. *Clinical Practice Guidelines in Oncology (NCCN Guidelines)*. Merkel Cell Carcinoma. Version 1.2021—February 18, 2021.
5. Lachance, K, Akaike T, Cahill K, et al. Detecting Merkel cell carcinoma recurrence using a blood test: outcomes from 774 patients. *J Investig Dermatol*. 2019;139(5):S101.

8

Rare Cancer Presentations

**Bilal Fawaz, Heather A. Edwards, Monica Rosales Santillan,
Debjani Sahni, Connor O'Boyle, and Daniel L. Faden**

CONTENTS

Case 8.1

Authors: Bilal Fawaz, MD, and Heather A. Edwards, MD.

Reason for Presentation: Diagnosis and management of a rare cutaneous malignancy.

Chief Complaint: Large growth on the scalp.

History of Present Illness: A middle-aged patient presented with a 19-year history of a growth on the scalp. The lesion initially started as a small, asymptomatic bump with gradual enlargement over this time. The lesions recurred after each of the three attempts at surgical removal at an outside institute. There was no history of having received prior chemotherapy or radiation. A rapid expansion and ulceration of the mass occurred 6 months prior to presentation to our cutaneous oncology clinic, which was approximately 2 years following the most recent excision.

Review of Systems: No pertinent positives.

Medical/Surgical History: None.

Medications: None.

Family History: No family history of skin cancer.

Social History: Denied tobacco, alcohol, or illicit drug use.

Physical Examination: Occipital scalp: Solitary 15×15 cm, exophytic, multi-lobulated tumor with a central large ulcer (Figure 8.1.1); Right submandibular region: 1 cm firm, rubbery, tender subcutaneous nodule; Cervical and axillary region without any palpable lymphadenopathy.

Pathology: Incisional biopsy of the occipital scalp tumor (Figure 8.1.2): (a) Large nodular tumor in the dermis with multiple areas of necrosis; (b) the tumor is composed of pale staining squamous epithelium with foci of trichilemmal keratinization; and (c) sheets of atypical epithelial cells with scattered mitoses.

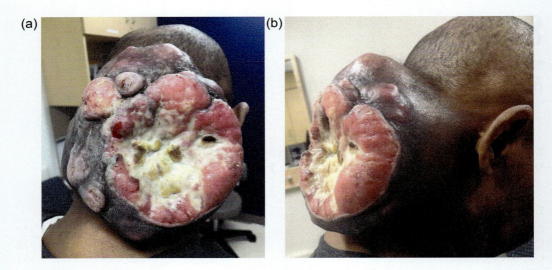

FIGURE 8.1.1   Large, exophytic, multi-lobulated tumor with focal areas of ulceration and white-yellow crust on the occipital scalp: (a) posterior view and (b) lateral view.

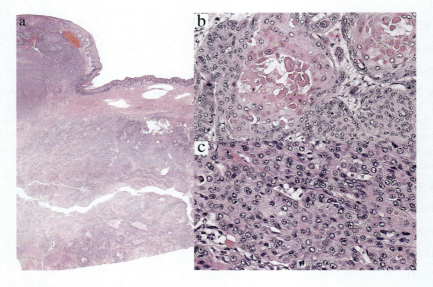

FIGURE 8.1.2   Incisional biopsy of the tumor on the occipital scalp: (a) H&E, 10×; (b) H&E, 300×; and (c) H&E, 300×.

Investigations

- **MRI cervical spine without contrast:** Large posterior cervical spine soft tissue lesion approximately measuring $14 \times 16 \times 10$ cm reaching but not involving the spinal canal. There is involvement of the paraspinal muscles but no definite bone involvement.
- **CT head and neck:** Large suboccipital ulcerating soft tissue mass measuring up to 14 cm with associated extensive cervical lymphadenopathy. There is suggestion of extension into the posterior epidural space between the occiput and C1. No obvious evidence for bone invasion.
- **CT chest, abdomen, and pelvis:** No evidence of metastatic disease.

Final Diagnosis: Malignant proliferating trichilemmal tumor (MPTT).

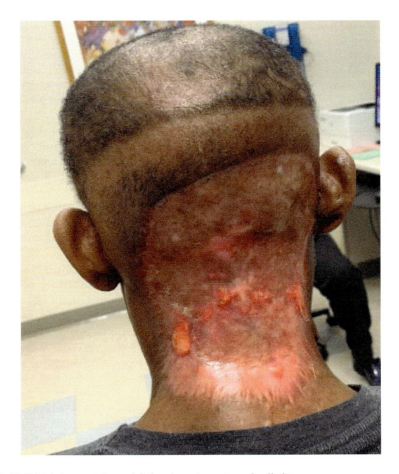

FIGURE 8.1.3 Well-healed scar on the occipital scalp post-surgery and radiation.

Management and Disease Course: A wide local excision, bilateral neck dissection, and flap reconstruction were performed. Resection margins were negative, and examination of the excised nodes found no evidence of metastatic disease. The patient's disease course was complicated by a post-operative wound infection, necessitating taking down the flap and letting it heal by secondary intention.

Adjuvant radiation within 6 weeks of surgery was recommended by the multidisciplinary tumor board due the tumor's extensive local invasion and high risk of recurrence. Given its proximity to the brainstem and spinal cord, conservative radiation was pursued to minimize the risk of deleterious neurologic adverse events secondary to treatment. The patient completed 6 weeks of radiotherapy with a total delivered dose of 60 Gy, and remains without evidence of recurrence to date 2 years post-treatment (Figure 8.1.3).

Discussion

- Trichilemmal cyst (TC), also known as pilar cyst, is a common, benign cyst originating from the outer root sheath of the hair follicle. Proliferating trichilemmal tumor (PTT) and its malignant counterpart MPTT are thought to arise from TC and are exceedingly rare.[1] The three neoplasms lie on a continuum with progressively worsening clinical behavior, histologic atypia, and architectural disorder.[2,3]
- The majority of TCs present as small, smooth, round, intradermal nodules on the scalp, most commonly in women over 40 years of age.[1] PTT/MPTT arise at similar locations but typically

undergo slow enlargement into exophytic masses with or without ulceration. They tend to range from 1 to 10 cm in size, but tumors as large as 25 cm have been reported.[1–3] PTT's clinical course ranges from indolent growth and high surgical cure rate to locally aggressive behavior with a high tendency for recurrence. MPTT specifically has the potential to metastasize to regional lymph nodes and distant sites, with studies suggesting a metastatic rate as high as 25% in high-grade MPTT.[1,3] Metastases have been shown to occur both at initial presentation or as late as 10 years post-diagnosis.[1]

- The histological hallmark of all the trichilemmal neoplasms is an abrupt transition of the nucleated epithelium to anucleated keratinized cells without a granular layer.[3] When cytologic atypia and architectural disorder are present, the diagnosis of PTT or MPTT is made. Considerable debate exists regarding the definition of benign versus malignant PTT. Following the largest study to date, Ye et al. proposed the separation of PTT and MPTT into three histologic groups (PTT, low-grade MPTT, high-grade MPTT) to estimate the risk of aggressive tumor behavior[3]:

  - **PPT:** Benign behaving lesions without recurrence; display well-circumscribed margins, modest nuclear atypia, with absence of pathologic mitoses, necrosis, or neurovascular invasion
  - **Low-grade MPTT:** Potential for recurrence and locally aggressive behavior; exhibits irregular, invasive margins and involves the deep dermis and subcutis
  - **High-grade MPTT:** Significant risk of recurrence and/or metastasis; manifest invasive patterns of growth; have marked nuclear atypia, pathologic mitotic forms, and geographic necrosis, with or without involvement of neurovascular structures

- The diagnosis of PTT/MPTT is often difficult to distinguish from SCC due to their significant histologic overlap. Immunohistochemical staining for pilar-type polypeptides, such as AE13 and AE14, are a useful tool in distinguishing between the entities. Most PTT stain positively with AE13 and AE14, while SCC are typically negative.[1]

- Given the rarity of this tumor, there are no NCCN guidelines to aid with management. Wide local excision with at least 1 cm margin and tumor clearance is the mainstay of treatment. Nodal dissection and adjuvant radiation should also be considered based on clinicopathologic features, extent of local spread and margin clearance. Mohs micrographic surgery provides superior margin control and may be considered where the surgeon feels comfortable with assessing the tissue pathology. Chemotherapy has shown limited success to date.[2]

Teaching Pearls

- PTT and MPTT lie on a continuum and are thought to originate from TC.
- Careful histologic examination is crucial in differentiating PTT from either low-or high-grade MPTT. The latter can be locally aggressive with a significantly high rate of recurrence and metastasis.
- Surgical treatment is first line for MPTT. Wide local excision with confirmation of histological margin clearance is most often utilized. Nodal dissection and adjuvant radiation should also be considered on a case-by-case basis dependent on the degree of spread.

References

1. Satyaprakash A, Sheehan D, Sangueza O. Proliferating trichilemmal tumors: a review of the literature. *Dermatol Surg.* 2007;33:1102–8.
2. Fieleke DR, Goldstein G. Malignant proliferating trichilemmal tumor treated with Mohs surgery: proposed protocol for diagnostic work-up and treatment. *Dermatol Surg.* 2015;41(2)292–94.
3. Ye J, Nappi O, Swanson P, et al. Proliferating pilar tumors. A clinicopathologic study of 76 cases with a proposal for definition of benign and malignant variants. *Am J Clin Pathol.* 2004;122:566–74.

Case 8.2

Authors: Monica Rosales Santillan, MD, Bilal Fawaz, MD, and Debjani Sahni, MD.

Reason for Presentation: Widespread and advanced basosquamous carcinoma and cutaneous squamous cell carcinoma in a patient with prior multiple unsuccessful attempts at surgery and radiation.

Chief Complaint: Numerous disfiguring growths on the face and arms.

History of Present Illness: A middle-aged patient with a history of multiple non-melanoma skin cancers (NMSCs) presented with a 3-year history of innumerable ulcerating growths on the nose, cheeks, and forearms. The patient had been previously managed in a country outside of the United States with several surgeries and sessions of radiation therapy in an attempt to clear the NMSCs. However, treatment was unsuccessful and the tumors had recurred.

Review of Systems: No pertinent positives.

Medical/Surgical History: Numerous NMSC on the face and arms, status post >15 surgical excisions and radiation therapy; the latter of unclear dose and duration.

Medications: None.

Family History: Father had skin cancer (not otherwise specified) on the nose.

Social History: Nil relevant.

Physical Examination: Skin type II; Face: Multiple crusted papules and nodules, in addition to nose—Large, ulcerated, crusted tumor with resulting destruction of underlying nasal cartilage and septum (Figure 8.2.1); Right cheek: 2.0 × 2.0 cm pink, ulcerated plaque with rolled borders and overlying crust; Left cheek: Large, pedunculated, hyperkeratotic tumor measuring approximately 4.0 × 2.0 × 2.0 cm; Bilateral upper limbs: Right lateral forearm—Hyperkeratotic, erythematous plaque; Left forearm—Multiple atrophic scars; large, fixed, tender left cervical adenopathy.

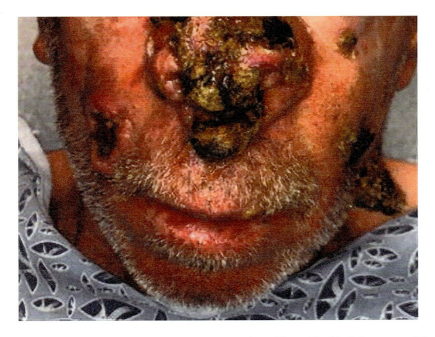

FIGURE 8.2.1   Numerous scattered crusted papulonodules on the face with considerable disfigurement of the nose; large hyperkeratotic tumor on the left jawline.

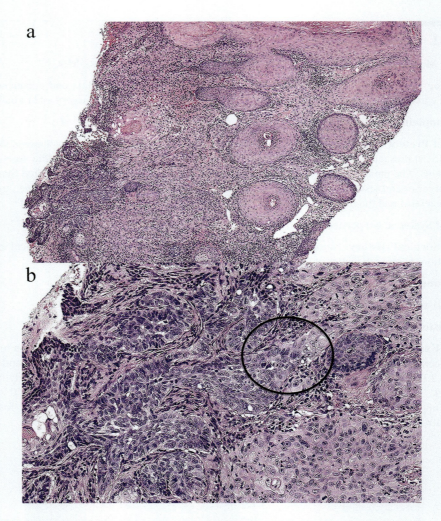

FIGURE 8.2.2 Punch biopsy of the right cheek: (a) H&E, 20× and (b) H&E, 200×.

Pathology: Punch biopsy of the right cheek nodule (Figure 8.2.2): (a) well-differentiated squamous cell carcinoma overlying and adjacent to a nodular and infiltrating basal cell carcinoma; (b) islands of basal cell carcinoma with retraction artifact (left) in continuity with atypical squamoid islands (right); punch biopsy of the right jawline: Acantholytic squamous cell carcinoma, well-differentiated.

Investigations

- **CT chest, neck with contrast:** Enhancing masses involving the nose, right cheek including deeper buccal soft tissues and the left cheek. A 2.5 cm enhancing lesion in the left parotid is non-specific metastatic adenopathy can be considered. Multiple 2–3 mm pulmonary nodules which are indeterminate. Correlation with patient's history of malignancy is recommended.
- **Left cervical lymph node FNA:** Positive for malignancy consistent with metastatic SCC.
- Gene mutation analysis from a skin biopsy sample of a basosquamous cell carcinoma (BSC) demonstrated a high somatic mutational burden (266 mutations/megabase) and 16 identified oncogenes or tumor suppressor gene mutations, several with multiple mutations/gene (*NOTCH2/3*, *PTCH1*, *SMO*, *TP53*, *CDKN2A*, and *MEN1*, among others).

Final Diagnosis: Multiple recurrent and locally advanced BSC and cutaneous squamous cell carcinoma (cSCC) with regional spread to the cervical lymph nodes; stage III (T3N1Mx).

Management and Disease Course: The multidisciplinary tumor board panel were faced with a very unusual and advanced presentation of multiple recurrent, high-risk NMSCs with evidence of regional metastasis, portending a poor prognosis. The clinical history and distribution of the tumors suggested the current presentation could be the result of inadequate tumor clearance of the NMSCs early on in treatment in addition to receiving multiple high doses of radiation. This allowed the tumors to relapse over time in previously scarred areas, making it progressively more difficult to clear the tumors, with ultimate spread of disease to the cervical nodes. The patient was otherwise in good health with no co morbidities. They were not of advanced age, and they were significantly cosmetically disfigured by the presentation. The management approach of the tumor board was to utilize various treatment modalities in sync (though not radiation) to improve the clinical presentation and overall quality of life for the patient, with the goal of long-term palliation if unable to achieve a cure.

Given the widespread, advanced nature of the NMSCs with evidence of metastasis, a PD-1 inhibitor was started at the outset, pembrolizumab (200 mg IV every 3 weeks), as this agent has been approved in a tissue-type agnostic manner for tumors with a high somatic mutation burden (>10 mutations/megabase). A slow partial response was noted. Based on data on the use of hedgehog pathway inhibitors in basosquamous tumors, vismodegib was then added to the regimen (150 mg daily). Combination systemic therapy resulted in ~50% reduction in tumor size within months, most notably on the nose and left cheek. There was also visible regrowth of healthy granulation tissue on the nasal septum. Side effects of mild-to-moderate dysgeusia secondary to vismodegib developed after a couple of months. Weakness in the right shoulder and contractures involving the right fourth and fifth fingers also evolved with treatment. The latter was thought to occur due to an immune-mediated brachial plexus neuritis. The side effects were tolerable to the patient, and importantly, their quality of life improved significantly. Surgical excision was utilized to debulk a large pedunculated tumor on the left cheek (which subsequently resolved with continued systemic therapy). The tender left cervical node was also removed surgically and further serial imaging did not show evidence of regional disease recurrence or new distant metastases over the following year.

After 6 months of treatment, the dysgeusia became more pronounced. Additionally, there was concern for the likely future development of drug resistance to vismodegib if this was continued long-term. At this point, the combination of treatment modalities had resulted in significant reduction in the size of the tumors with a plateau in tumor response. Given this, vismodegib was discontinued (with return of normal taste), but the PD-1 inhibitor therapy was continued given the persistence of active disease. The lesions remained stable off vismodegib at a 6-month follow-up visit (Figure 8.2.3). The patient was referred for Mohs micrographic surgery to remove any persistent clinical lesions (which were now much smaller in size). A referral was also made to head and neck surgery for a prosthetic nose.

Discussion

- Patients with exposure to ionizing radiation therapy (RT) have an increased risk of NMSC, most commonly basal cell carcinomas, followed by SCCs.[1,2] The majority of cases develop within previously irradiated fields after a median latency of 15–20 years (range 2–65 years), with shorter incubation periods in younger patients.[1,2]

- A recent study of 86 Hodgkin's lymphoma patients demonstrated a standardized incidence ratio of 15.9 (95% CI: 9.1–25.9) in secondary skin cancers in RT patients with long-term follow-up, resulting in 626 excess cases per 10,000 patients per year.[1] When compared to chemotherapy, RT significantly increased the risk of skin cancer development, with a hazard ratio of 2.75 (95% CI: 1.01–7.45).[1] Ionizing radiation is thought to directly induce DNA damage and promote cell migration through reactive oxygen species formation, thereby increasing the risk of secondary malignancies.[3]

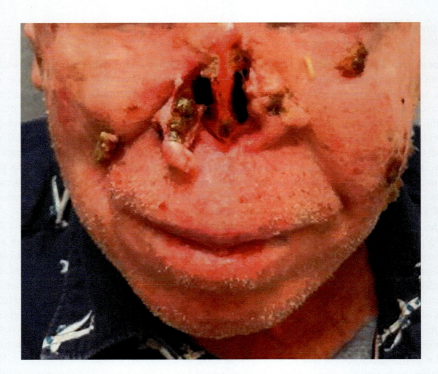

FIGURE 8.2.3   Clinical resolution of multiple lesions on the face. The residual tumors show significant reduction in size compared to the initial visit.

- BSC is a hybrid neoplasm characterized histologically by the presence of both BCC and SCC features, along with an intermediary transition zone.[4] While the clinical presentation overlaps with other NMSCs, the behavior of BSC is considered to be more aggressive, with higher rates of local recurrence and distant metastasis when compared to its more common counterparts.[4,5]

- Several studies have analyzed the mutational burden in BSC to better understand its origin and pathogenesis.[5,6] A recent study by Chiang et al. demonstrated early PTCH1 or SMO mutations in the majority of BSCs, as well as a lack of common SCC driver mutations (such as *NOTCH1* and *NOTCH2*).[5] These early changes were followed by subsequent mutations involving the RAS-MAPK pathway, which are involved in SCC development.[5] The findings support the theory that BSC originally derives from BCC, followed by additional mutations that result in their squamatization.[5]

- The current treatment of choice for BSC is surgical management with Mohs micrographic surgery.[6] Medical management has not been well-established due to tumor rarity. Vismodegib, which is FDA-approved for advanced BCC, has been reported to be effective in treating BSC, although data are limited.[7] In a case series involving two patients, vismodegib was initiated in non-surgical candidates, resulting in complete response by 7 months and no recurrence at 9 months post-treatment.[7]

- Similarly, no studies currently exist on immunotherapy for the treatment of BSC. However, the efficacy of PD-1 inhibitors in NMSC treatment, coupled with our patient's high somatic mutational burden, led us to hypothesize that our patient may similarly respond to pembrolizumab.[8]

Teaching Pearls

- Exposure to ionizing radiation increases the risk of NMSCs (BCC > SCC) after a median latency of 15–20 years (range 2–65 years).
- BSC is an aggressive subtype of NMSC with an increased risk of local recurrence and distant metastasis.
- While surgical management remains first line, vismodegib and/or PD-1 inhibitors may be considered in non-surgical candidates, though more studies are needed to support this clinical approach.

References

1. Daniëls LA, Krol AD, Schaapveld M, et al. Long-term risk of secondary skin cancers after radiation therapy for Hodgkin's lymphoma. *Radiother Oncol*. 2013;109(1):140–5.
2. Marín-Gutzke M, Sánchez-Olaso A, Berenguer B, et al. Basal cell carcinoma in childhood after radiation therapy: case report and review. *Ann Plast Surg*. 2004;53(6):593–5.
3. Lee SY, Jeong EK, Ju MK, et al. Induction of metastasis, cancer stem cell phenotype, and oncogenic metabolism in cancer cells by ionizing radiation. *Mol Cancer*. 2017;16(1):10.
4. Tan CZ, Rieger KE, Sarin KY. Basosquamous carcinoma: controversy, advances, and future directions. *Dermatol Surg*. 2017;43(1):23–31.
5. Chiang A, Tan CZ, Kuonen F, et al. Genetic mutations underlying phenotypic plasticity in basosquamous carcinoma. *J Invest Dermatol*. 2019;139(11):2263–71.
6. Wermker K, Roknic N, Goessling K, et al. Basosquamous carcinoma of the head and neck: clinical and histologic characteristics and their impact on disease progression. *Neoplasia*. 2015;17(3):301–5.
7. Apalla Z, Giakouvis V, Gavros Z, et al. Complete response of locally advanced basosquamous carcinoma to vismodegib in two patients. *Eur J Dermatol*. 2019;29(1):102–4.
8. Lipson EJ, Lilo MT, Ogurtsova A, et al. Basal cell carcinoma: PD-L1/PD-1 checkpoint expression and tumor regression after PD-1 blockade. *J Immunother Cancer*. 2017;21:5–23.

Case 8.3

Authors: Connor O'Boyle, BS, Bilal Fawaz, MD, and Daniel L. Faden, MD, FACS.

Reason for Presentation: Rare presentation of a deep fibrous histiocytoma (FH).

Chief Complaint: Growth on the left cheek.

History of Present Illness: A young adult presented with a 6-month history of a painful growth on the left cheek. The lesion initially started as a "bump below the skin" with a more rapid increase in size in the weeks prior to presentation. The patient denied any associated drainage or pruritus.

Review of Systems: No pertinent positives.

Medical/Surgical History: Nil relevant.

Medications: None.

Family History: No family history of skin cancer.

Social History: Five-pack-year history of smoking cigarettes.

Physical Examination: Left malar cheek: Ill-defined dermal swelling on the left cheek with multi-lobulated, firm, fixed induration on palpation (Figure 8.3.1).

Pathology: Incisional biopsy of the left zygoma tumor (Figure 8.3.2): A spindle-cell tumor with focal necrosis exhibiting a storiform and herringbone pattern, infiltrating dermal collagen, and focally extending into skeletal muscle. Immunoperoxidase staining demonstrates multifocal positivity of the lesional cells with CD34 and SMA. Subsequent excision of the left facial tumor demonstrated a cellular, spindle-cell neoplasm with multifocal positivity for SMA and epithelial membrane antigen (EMA). Immunoperoxidase stains were negative for CD34, ERG, and PAN-TRK. No rearrangement of the *PDGFB* gene region was detected on FISH.

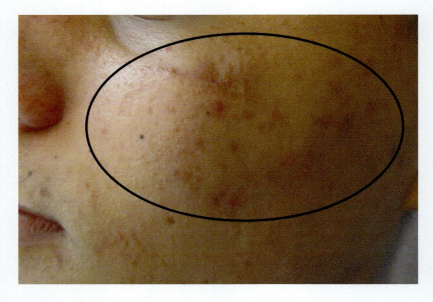

FIGURE 8.3.1   Ill-defined dermal swelling on the left cheek with multi-lobulated, firm, fixed induration on palpation.

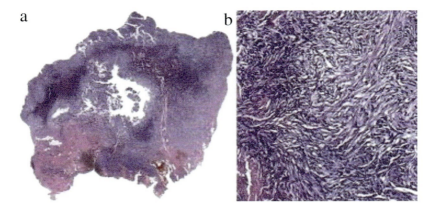

FIGURE 8.3.2   Incisional biopsy of the left cheek tumor: (a) H&E, low power and (b) H&E, high power.

Investigations

- MRI neck with and without contrast: A 2.2 cm mass extending from the skin to the left zygoma. There is involvement of the underlying muscles of facial expression including the left orbicularis oculi and the left zygomaticus muscles. No evidence of underlying bone marrow involvement or underlying cortical destruction of the zygoma.

Diagnosis: Deep FH.

Management and Disease Course: The patient was taken to the operating room for planned staged resection and reconstruction by the head and neck surgical oncology team. Initial resection included skin of the face and facial musculature down to the level of the facial skeleton with 1 cm margins circumferentially and 0.8 cm margins cranially to avoid the eyelid skin. The tumor was found to be attached to the periosteum of the zygoma and inferior orbital rim and wrapping behind the maxilla into the pterygomaxillary fissure. The tumor was cleared en bloc and the cortical bone of the inferior orbital rim and zygoma were burred down, margins were sent circumferentially from the skin and deep tissues for permanent evaluation. The wound was packed, and a second stage resection and reconstruction were planned for the following week.

Pathology confirmed deep fibrous histiocytoma with positive margins laterally. Lateral margins were re-resected and reconstruction performed with a radial forearm free flap, temporalis tendon transfer, and canthopexy (Figure 8.3.3). The case was discussed at tumor board including whether to advise adjuvant radiation. In the end, the tumor board panel decided to forego adjuvant radiation as its efficacy is largely unknown in the setting of deep FH. Additionally, the long-term side effects from radiation at the tumor location (keratoconjunctivitis sicca, cataracts) and risk for secondary malignancy (radiation-induced sarcoma) in a young patient were felt to outweigh the benefits. Instead, active surveillance was advised including clinical examination every 3 months and serial MRI scan every 6 months. The patient remains disease-free 3 years post-surgery.

Discussion

- Benign FH or dermatofibroma are common mesenchymal tumors of the skin. Various histological variants have been described (e.g., epithelial, palisading, cellular, atypical) some with distinct clinical features such as propensity for local recurrence, for example, cellular FH. Most FH are cutaneous in origin, but a small subset ~5% arise in subcutaneous or deep soft tissue and are termed deep FH (DFH).[1] DFH often present as a solitary, firm, non-mobile, painless dermal nodule, ranging from 0.5 to 25 cm in size.[1–3] It most commonly arises on an extremity (58%–80% of cases), followed by the head/neck (14%–22%) and trunk (6%–11%).[1,2]

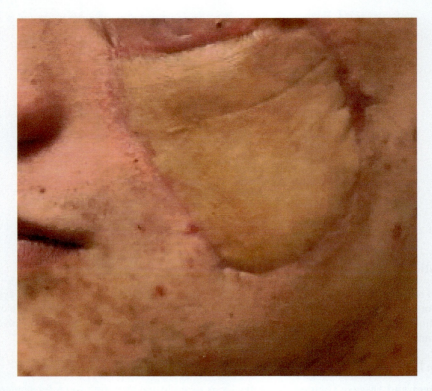

FIGURE 8.3.3   Well-healed surgical site following wide local excision and reconstruction on the left cheek.

- Histologically, DFH is a well-circumscribed subcutaneous spindle-cell neoplasm with a thick fibrous pseudo-capsule. It displays a storiform pattern of plump spindle cells with intermixed lymphocytes and entrapment of collagen bundles, in addition to a fascicular growth pattern with frequent extension into subcutaneous tissue. Foam cells, multinucleate giant cells, including Touton giant cells, and osteoclastic giant cells have also been reported. Immunohistochemical staining can demonstrate positivity for Factor XIIIa, CD34, and smooth muscle actin; it is sometimes focally positive for desmin. Staining is often negative for EMA.[1,2]

- The differential diagnoses for DFH include solitary fibrous tumor, dermatofibrosarcoma protuberans (DFSP), and undifferentiated pleomorphic sarcoma (UPS).[1] Significant clinical overlap exists between these entities as they typically present as painless, non-mobile, subcutaneous nodules. Histologically, DFH has a storiform pattern and uniform cellularity, while solitary fibrous tumor is defined by a "patternless" architecture. UPS is characterized by a high mitotic count with cellular pleomorphism.[2]

- Differentiating DFSP and DFH can be difficult as both have a storiform architecture. DFH invades surrounding tissue with a smooth, pushing border, unlike DFSP, which invades surrounding tissues through tentacle-like projections from a central tumor focus. Immunohistochemical staining of DFSP also reveals CD34 positivity in 50%–100% of reactive cells, while DFH only shows focal reactivity with less than 20% of cells.[1] Given the considerable clinicopathologic overlap between both entities, genetic testing for the t(17;22) translocation may be considered in diagnostically challenging cases as the pathogenesis of both tumors is different. The t(17;22) is only positive in DFSP.[2] The translocation results in the fusion of the COL1A1 gene from chromosome 17 with the PDGFB gene from chromosome 22, resulting in uncontrolled cellular proliferation and growth.[2]

- Treatment for DFH involves wide local excision with the most commonly cited margins being 1–2 cm, although no consensus has been reached.[5,6] As with all facial surgeries, margins are frequently modified to preserve critical anatomic structure and subunits. There is a paucity of data on the efficacy of radiation or chemotherapy in treating DFH.[2–4]

- Long-term follow-up is essential due to the relatively high local recurrence rates in up to 22% of cases.[2–4] Recurrence is more common in men and in large tumors (initial size >1 cm).[1,2] Five percent of patients with DFH (2/69 in the Gleason and Fletcher study) developed metastasis, and both ultimately died of their disease. This may be an overestimation of the likelihood of metastasis due to inherent selection (referral) bias. Histologically, there were no significant differences between metastasizing and non-metastasizing primary tumors.[2]

- DFH of the face is particularly associated with infiltration of the subcutaneous and deep soft tissue, including striated muscle, due to the limited soft tissue depth of the face.[3] As a result of this infiltrative tendency and possible hesitancy to complete wide local excisions that necessitate functional reconstruction, higher recurrence rates have been associated with DFH of the face.[3]

Teaching Pearls

- DFH is a rare subtype of benign FH (dermatofibroma). It classically presents as a solitary, hard, non-mobile, painless nodule on an extremity, though it can also occur in the head/neck region.

- Differential diagnoses include dermatofibroma sarcoma protuberans, solitary fibrous tumors and UPS.

- The treatment of choice is surgical excision ensuring clear margins. Close follow-up is recommended due to high local recurrence rates and rarely the possibility of metastasis. There is very limited data on the efficacy of chemotherapy and radiation for this entity.

References

1. Gaufin M, Michaelis T, Duffy K. Cellular dermatofibroma: clinicopathologic review of 218 cases of cellular dermatofibroma to determine the clinical recurrence rate. *Dermatol Surg.* 2019;45(11). doi:10.1097/DSS.0000000000001833.
2. Gleason BC, Fletcher CDM. Deep "benign" fibrous histiocytoma: clinicopathologic analysis of 69 cases of a rare tumor indicating occasional metastatic potential. *Am J Surg Pathol.* 2008;32(3). doi:10.1097/PAS.0b013e31813c6b85.
3. Mentzel T, Kutzner H, Rütten A, et al. Benign fibrous histiocytoma (dermatofibroma) of the face: clinicopathologic and immunohistochemical study of 34 cases associated with an aggressive clinical course. *Am J Dermatotopathol.* 2001;23(5):419–26. doi:10.1097/00000372-200110000-00006.
4. Chung J, Namkoong S, Sim JH, et al. Deep penetrating benign fibrous histiocytoma of the foot associated with throbbing pain. *Ann Dermatol.* 2011;23(suppl. 2):S239–42. doi:10.5021/ad.2011.23.S2.S239.
5. Arikanoglu Z, Akbulut S, Basbug M, et al. Benign fibrous histiocytoma arising from the intercostal space. *General Thorac Cardiovasc Surg.* 2011;59(11):763–6. doi:10.1007/s11748-010-0760-2.
6. Akbulut S, Arikanoglu Z, Basbug M. Benign fibrous histiocytoma arising from the right shoulder: is immunohistochemical staining always required for a definitive diagnosis? *Int J Surg Case Rep.* 2012;3(7):287–9.

Index

Bold page numbers refer to tables; *italic* page numbers refer to figures.